Evidence-Based Practice in Nursing

A GUIDE TO SUCCESSFUL IMPLEMENTATION

Suzanne C. Beyea, RN, PhD, FAAN

Mary Jo Slattery, RN, MS

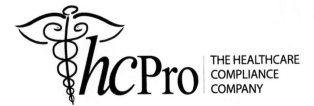

THE HEALTHCARE
COMPLIANCE
COMPANY

Evidence-Based Practice in Nursing: A Guide to Successful Implementation is published by HCPro, Inc.

HCPro, Inc., provides information resources for the healthcare industry.

MAGNET™, MAGNET RECOGNITION PROGRAM®, and ANCC MAGNET RECOGNITION® are trademarks of the American Nurses Credentialing Center (ANCC). The products and services of HCPro, Inc. and The Greeley Company are neither sponsored nor endorsed by the ANCC. The acronym "MRP" is not a trademark of HCPro or its parent company.

Suzanne C. Beyea, RN, PhD, FAAN, Author
Mary Jo Slattery, RN, MS, Author
Julie Shocksnider, RNC, MS, CCE, Contributing Author
Marian C. Turkel, RN, PhD, Contributor
Rebecca Hendren, Senior Managing Editor
Patrick Campagnone, Cover Designer

Lauren Rubenzahl, Copy Editor
Jackie Diehl Singer, Graphic Artist
Jean St. Pierre, Director of Operations
Emily Sheahan, Group Publisher
Paul Singer, Layout Artist

Advice given is general. Readers should consult professional counsel for specific legal, ethical, or clinical questions. Arrangements can be made for quantity discounts. For more information, contact

HCPro, Inc.
200 Hoods Lane
P.O. Box 1168
Marblehead, MA 01945
Telephone: 800/650-6787 or 781/639-1872
Fax: 781/639-2982
E-mail: *customerservice@hcpro.com*

Visit HCPro, Inc., at its World Wide Web sites: *www.hcpro.com* and *www.hcmarketplace.com*

Rev. 09/2007
21277

Contents

Contents

Acknowledgments

I would like to acknowledge my colleagues and students from the past three decades. These individuals have influenced my thinking about and practice of nursing research and my awareness of the need to ensure professional practice environments in which evidence-based practice can flourish. My sincerest thanks to my Dartmouth-Hitchcock Medical Center colleagues, past and present, who value and actualize evidence-based practice in practice, education, and leadership. Working in an organization with a long tradition of promoting nursing excellence shows me how evidence-based practice and high-quality patient care occur synergistically.

Writing takes time, resources, and the special efforts of a dedicated team. I extend my heartfelt gratitude to Elizabeth Cooper and Chris Parker, who reviewed drafts and provided careful and thoughtful edits under a fairly demanding timeline. Both my co-author, Mary Jo Slattery, and contributing author, Julie Shocksnider, must be thanked for their excellent contributions and recognized for their commitment to both their profession and evidence-based practice. My special thanks to Nancy A. Formella, senior nurse executive, and Linda J. Kobokovich, director of nursing practice and administration, for their support on this particular effort and many others. I must also acknowledge the Matthew-Fuller Library librarians and staff, who seamlessly provide electronic library resources to our entire organization as well as ongoing support for evidence-based practice. The team at HCPro, specifically Rebecca Hendren, has provided invaluable support and has been willing to help at every step of the process.

My sincerest thanks to my life partner and spouse, George, who supports my commitment to the profession of nursing and the sometimes endless hours I commit to various professional activities. I offer a special acknowledgement to Dr. Annette Beyea, who has brought joy to my life and work. Her integration of evidence-based practice in the care of her patients provides inspiration to my work. Lastly, I would like to acknowledge my family members and friends, for whom I have always wanted the very best in evidence-based care.

—Suzanne C. Beyea, RN, PhD, FAAN

Acknowledgments

I would like to express my deepest gratitude to my co-author, Suzanne Beyea, for her wisdom, friendship, and mentorship in writing this book. I sincerely appreciate her helping me see what is possible.

I would like to acknowledge all of my nursing colleagues, near and far, who have taught me so much about nursing research and evidence-based practice. I would especially like to thank all the Dartmouth-Hitchcock Medical Center nurses who have included me in their research, research utilization, and evidence-based practice projects over the past 15 years. I am truly inspired by their passion for asking the right questions and their commitment to providing the highest-quality patient care.

This project would not have been possible were it not for an environment that fosters a commitment to professional nursing practice. I wish to acknowledge Nancy Formella, senior nurse executive, and Linda Kobokovich, director of nursing practice and administration, for their dynamic leadership and support.

I would like to recognize all of the staff in the Office of Professional Nursing for their contributions to the project. I would especially like to thank Liz Cooper for her patience, good humor, and thoughtful reviews of this manuscript.

Finally, I would like to thank my husband, Andy, for his unending support and encouragement of this and other projects.

—Mary Jo Slattery, RN, MS

Suzanne C. Beyea, RN, PhD, FAAN

Suzanne C. Beyea, RN, PhD, FAAN, is the Director of Nursing Research at the Dartmouth-Hitchcock Medical Center (DHMC) in Lebanon, NH. Her responsibilities include supporting evidence-based practice, developing the clinical nursing research program for the medical center, and supporting nurses' efforts to use or conduct research. Her activities include providing consultation, education, technical support, and advice related to research, evidence-based practice, and the evaluation of nursing practices and clinical processes. She also serves as the ANCC Magnet Recognition Program® coordinator.

Beyea's nursing publications include journal articles, contributions to textbooks, and monthly columns on research topics and patient safety issues for the *AORN Journal.* She also has numerous publications related to the care of the medical-surgical patient, structured vocabulary, geriatric issues, and patient safety. In addition, she has extensive experience presenting educational sessions related to research, evidence-based practice, best practice, clinical competence, clinical pathways, care of the elderly client, quality improvement and outcomes management, using the clinical value compass to achieve best practices, legal aspects of documentation, and human patient simulation. Currently, she is the primary investigator for an HRSA-funded project called "Nurse Residency Program for Competency Development." She is actively involved in numerous local, regional, and national nursing organizations.

Mary Jo Slattery, RN, MS

Mary Jo Slattery, RN, MS, is the Nursing Research Coordinator at DHMC. She collaborates with the Director of Nursing Research, Suzanne Beyea, in the Office of Professional Nursing to support and facilitate research and evidence-based practice efforts in nursing. Her activities include consulting for and assisting with groups and individuals on such topics as online searching, project planning, instrument development, obtaining Institutional Review Board (IRB) approval, data collection, data analysis, and report writing. She manages the departmental review for nursing research studies prior to submission to the IRB and coordinates the use of statistical analysis software and conducts analysis on selected projects.

Slattery has more than 15 years of experience working with staff nurses in the acute care setting in conducting and using research, and most recently, in evidence-based practice. She is also involved in several professional nursing projects in the institution. She was co-principle investigator on a DHMC Quality Research Grant funded project "Evaluation of the Effectiveness of a Targeted Ergonomic Program to Prevent Back and Other Musculoskeletal Injuries in Nursing Personnel." Currently, she is the NDNQI Site Coordinator and the data manager and analyst on the HRSA-funded project "Nurse Residency Program for Competency Development."

Contributing author: Julie Shocksnider, RNC, MS, CCE

Julie Shocksnider, RNC, MS, CCE, is the Perinatal Clinical Nurse Specialist at DHMC. She received her Master of Science with her focus in nursing as a Perinatal Nurse Practitioner and Maternal/Child Clinical Nurse Specialist from Rutgers, the State University of New Jersey, and her Bachelor of Science in Nursing from the University of Louisville, KY. She has helped develop evidence-based nursing practice activities and previously chaired a nursing research committee. She has spoken about nurses' perceptions of nursing research and continues to be interested and involved in research practice activities.

What is evidence-based practice?

Learning objectives

After reading this chapter, the participant should be able to
- define evidence-based practice (EBP)
- differentiate between evidence-based practice, research, research utilization, and quality improvement
- describe the importance of EBP to nursing practice and high-quality patient care

Evidence-based practice

During the 1980s, the term "evidence-based medicine" emerged to describe the approach that used scientific evidence to determine the best practice. Later, the term shifted to become "evidence-based practice" as clinicians other than physicians recognized the importance of scientific evidence in clinical decision-making. Various definitions of evidence-based practice (EBP) have emerged in the literature, but the most commonly used definition is, "the conscientious, explicit, and judicious use of the current best evidence in making decisions about the care of individual patients" (Sackett, Rosenberg, Gray, Hayes, & Richardson, 1996).

Subsequently, experts began to talk about evidence-based healthcare as a process by which research evidence is used in making decisions about a specific population or group of patients. Evidence-based practice and evidence-based healthcare assume that evidence is used in the context of a particular patient's preferences and desires, the clinical situation, and the expertise of the clinician. They also expect that healthcare professionals can read, critique, and synthesize research findings and interpret existing evidence-based clinical practice guidelines.

Nurses ask numerous questions when looking to integrate evidence-based practice into their clinical environment:

- What exactly is EBP?
- Is EBP the same as nursing research?
- What is the difference between EBP and quality improvement?
- Is EBP relevant to nursing practice?

This book examines EBP and demonstrates its relevance to professional nursing practice and high-quality patient care.

Definitions of research utilization, quality improvement, and nursing research

Evidence-based practice is not research utilization, quality improvement, or nursing research, although it may be related to each of these processes. For example, quality improvement projects may be evidence-based, and the findings may contribute to other EBP or research initiatives. Also, an evidence-based practice project can lead to a research study or quality improvement initiative.

What is research utilization?

For decades, nurses have used available research to guide nursing practice and their efforts to improve patient outcomes. This process involved critical analysis and evaluation of research findings and then determining how they fit into clinical practice. Incorporating pertinent research findings into clinical practice (and evaluating the changes' effectiveness), helps close the gap between research and practice.

More recently, research utilization efforts in nursing have been replaced by evidence-based practice, which will be described in further detail later in this chapter.

What is quality or performance improvement?

Quality, clinical, or performance improvement focuses on systems, processes, and functional, clinical, satisfaction, and cost outcomes. Typically, quality improvement efforts are not designed to develop nursing practice standards or nursing science, but they may contribute to understanding best practices or the processes of care in which nurses are actively involved.

A commonly accepted view is that quality improvement activities in healthcare are not intended to generate scientific knowledge but rather to serve as management tools to improve the processes and outcomes within a specific healthcare organization or setting. More recently, experts have focused on improving care by examining and working within clinical microsystems or the specific places where patients, families, and care teams meet (Nelson, et al., 2002). To improve and maintain quality, safety, and efficiency, clinical teams must blend analysis, change, and measurement into their efforts to redesign care within these clinical microsystems.

Quality improvement initiatives generally address clinical problems or issues, examine clinical processes, and use specific indicators to help evaluate clinical performance. Data are collected and analyzed to help understand both the process and the related outcomes. The findings help contribute to efforts to achieve and maintain continuous improvement through ongoing monitoring and improvement activities.

For example, a hospital might be interested in improving its smoking cessation education for hospitalized patients, so it may convene a multidisciplinary team to address the issue. The team may decide to measure the hospital's performance using the percentage of discharge summaries that indicate that a smoker received instruction about smoking cessation. The team might implement an educational program and an electronic discharge summary that prompts clinicians to indicate whether the patient is a smoker and, if so, whether he or she received smoking cessation advice. They would monitor the rate of compliance and modify the interventions until compliance with the requirement to provide smoking cessation advice is greater than 95%.

Quality improvement projects vs. research projects

Many have asked whether quality improvement projects are the same as research projects—they are not. In clinical practice, these efforts may seem similar in that, for example, both may seek answers to clinical problems and use similar data collection and analysis methods. However, factors that may differ include participant or subject recruitment, the study's methods, and how the results are used.

For example, in most quality improvement activities, the participants generally are the patients within a specific clinical microsystem. In research efforts, the investigator recruits human subjects using approaches that will ensure a representative sample of the population. In many improvement activities, the intervention may change as it is evaluated, whereas in a research study the treatment or intervention remains the same.

Furthermore, in most quality improvement initiatives, the healthcare team is trying to solve a problem in a particular setting instead of trying to generalize the results of the study to other settings and populations. Although it might be helpful to learn about the activities and experience of other improvement teams, their findings may not apply to or be appropriate in other settings or patient populations. The intent of research, however, is to develop new knowledge that can be generalized to other similar populations and clinical settings.

Despite the differences between research and quality improvement projects, however, one must consider the protection of human subjects in both. To ensure that you adequately protect the rights of patients or subjects, always ask an Institutional Review Board (IRB) to review the research proposal or quality improvement project before implementing the study and beginning data collection.

Also note that, whether the effort is research or quality improvement, one goal may be to disseminate the results of the project in a published paper or oral report. For any dissemination project, address adequate human subject protection and adherence with the Health Information Portability and Accountability Act of 1996 (HIPAA) guidelines *before* beginning the improvement project or research study. Individuals involved in either quality improvement or research projects should seek advice from their organization's IRB, privacy officer, and risk management department to ensure that data are managed in a manner consistent with any pertinent federal or state regulations and organizational policies and procedures.

Examples of quality improvement projects

Sample quality improvement projects that have been conducted in healthcare organizations work to do the following:

- Reduce the time interval between when a provider writes an antibiotic order to when the patient receives the first dose

- Evaluate the effectiveness of a targeted ergonomic program to prevent injuries in nursing personnel

- Assess the effectiveness of a fast-track program on patient satisfaction in the emergency department

- Optimize the prevention and treatment of anemia during coronary artery bypass surgery

- Improve the care of patients with Type II diabetes using shared medical appointments

- Decrease blood stream infections associated with central venous catheters

- Improve adherence with recommendations for education about smoking cessation

- Improve and maintain adherence with core best practices in the intensive care unit

- Improve patient satisfaction through noise reduction activities

- Assess the effectiveness of using a fall-risk assessment in decreasing the number and severity of patient falls

The above example related to falls could also be an evidence-based practice or research project. If after searching the nursing literature you found another fall-risk assessment tool and you changed practice in your organization, the information you collected could contribute to an evidence-based project. You also might find multiple best practices or nursing interventions related to falls prevention. You can use this information to formulate a research question and conduct a nursing research study within your organization to see which interventions provide the best outcomes in your specific patient population.

Multidisciplinary efforts
Within clinical settings, many such opportunities exist for both nursing and multidisciplinary improvement efforts. Improvement activities for nursing can be as simple as reducing time in giving verbal report or improving compliance with documentation requirements. Multidisciplinary collaborative efforts may address complex health issues, such as the care of acute myocardial infarction patients or individuals with community-acquired pneumonia.

These initiatives are becoming more important in acute care hospitals as the national focus on public reporting increases. Such efforts help consumers compare the quality of care that various hospitals provide. The Centers for Medicare & Medicaid Services (CMS); various organizations that represent hospitals, doctors, and employers; accrediting organizations; other federal agencies; and the public have combined efforts to develop Hospital Compare (*www.hospitalcompare.hhs.gov*) and, thus, have made key clinical outcome measures available to the public. In this way, the public can monitor performance indicators to related common medical conditions and certain evidence-based interventions that are consistent with achieving the best patient outcomes.

Collaboration within multidisciplinary teams creates opportunities to address clinical problems and issues using various perspectives and expertise. Nurses play key roles in such efforts and often benefit from the synergy that can be realized by working with others interested in or concerned about the problem. For example, if an organization determines that patients are experiencing elevated blood sugars and not achieving good glucose control, a decision might be made to address this issue. Nurses alone can't solve this problem and need the support of physicians, dieticians, pharmacists, and perhaps other specialists. Bringing together a team of nurses, physicians, and other clinicians concerned about diabetic care provides opportunities for all members of the team to solve problems creatively. The group can work together while measuring their progress against pre-determined objectives.

What is nursing research?

Nursing research involves systematic inquiry specifically designed to develop, refine, and extend nursing knowledge. As part of a clinical and professional discipline, nurses have a unique body of knowledge that addresses nursing practice, administration, and education. Nurse researchers examine problems of specific concern to nurses and the patients, families, and communities they serve.

Nursing research methods may be quantitative, qualitative, or mixed (i.e., triangulated):

- In **quantitative studies**, researchers use objective, quantifiable data (such as blood pressure or pulse rate) or use a survey instrument to measure knowledge, attitudes, beliefs, or experiences

- **Qualitative researchers** use methods such as interviews or narrative analyses to help understand a particular phenomenon

- **Triangulated approaches** use both quantitative and qualitative methods

Regardless of the method they use, researchers must adhere to certain approaches to ensure both the quality and the accuracy of the data and related analyses. The intent of each approach is to answer questions and develop knowledge using the scientific method.

Examples of nursing research projects

Examples of nursing research projects include the following:

- Randomized clinical trial examining best practice for orthopedic-pin site care
- Efficacy of examination gloves for simple dressing changes
- Reliability of methods used to determine nasogastric tube placement
- The effects of relaxation and guided imagery on preoperative anxiety
- Quality of life in patients with chronic pain
- The relationship of a preoperative teaching program for joint replacement surgery and patient outcomes

The scientific method involves collecting observable, measurable, and verifiable data in a prescribed manner so as to describe, explain, or predict outcomes. For example, one might collect data to describe the effects of massage on blood pressure, explain decreased needs for sedation, or predict lower levels of anxiety.

Research methods demand that the collected data remain objective and not be influenced by the researcher's hypotheses, beliefs, or values. In the massage example, the researcher could easily bias the results by administering the massages or collecting the data. Using certain approaches to subject recruitment, performing faulty data collection, and not controlling for other confounding variables also can bias research findings. Therefore, when developing a study proposal, the researcher must develop a plan that minimizes these risks and supports the development of reliable information and results.

Conducting nursing research is not as simple as saying, "I want to do research." To conduct a scientific investigation, the researcher must have adequate training and resources. Developing and implementing a well-designed study with adequate control requires extensive knowledge of research methods and processes. Therefore, nurses interested in conducting research may work with an experienced researcher or develop their own skills by taking statistics and research methods courses and by being mentored by someone with research skills. One approach that staff nurses can take to get involved in research is to learn about and get involved in efforts related to evidence-based nursing practice. Working with others who have expertise in evidence-based practice serves as a helpful introduction into the processes of critiquing, analyzing, and evaluating published research, which is a necessary step in any research activity.

EBP implications for nurses

Nurses serve instrumental roles in ensuring and providing evidence-based practice. They must continually ask the questions, "What is the evidence for this intervention?" or "How do we provide best practice?" and "Are these the highest achievable outcomes for the patient, family, and nurse?" Nurses are also well positioned to work with other members of the healthcare team to identify clinical problems and use existing evidence to improve practice. Numerous opportunities exist for nurses to question current nursing practices and use evidence to make care more effective.

For example, a recently published evidence-based project describes the potential benefits of discontinuing the routine practice of listening to the bowel sounds of patients who have undergone elective abdominal surgery. The authors reviewed the literature and conducted an assessment of current practice, and they subsequently developed and evaluated a new practice guideline. These authors reported that clinical parameters such as the return of flatus and first postoperative bowel movement were more helpful than bowel sounds in determining the return of gastrointestinal mobility after abdominal surgery. The authors found that this evidence-based project resulted in saving nursing time without having negative patient outcomes (Madsen et al., 2005).

Nurses throughout the country also have been involved in multidisciplinary efforts to reduce the number and severity of falls and pressure ulcers/injuries. Such projects can help save money and improve care processes and outcomes. By implementing existing evidence-based guidelines related to falls and pressure ulcers/injuries, care has improved, and the number and severity of negative outcomes have decreased. Other examples of evidence-based healthcare efforts include projects to increase compliance with requirements for screenings for cancer and improving glucose control.

Importance of evidence-based practice

Evidence-based practice helps nurses provide high-quality patient care based on research and knowledge rather than because "this is the way we have always done it," or based on traditions, myths, hunches, advice of colleagues, or outdated textbooks.

For example, when clinical questions arise, should one look to a nursing textbook for the answers? Remember that books are not published every year, and new information may not be included in the edition you have. Also, when using textbooks, consider whether you have the most current edition. There are also issues to consider when asking colleagues for advice—specifically, be mindful that their responses may be based on their personal experiences, their observations, what they learned in school, what was reviewed during nursing orientation, or myths and traditions learned in clinical practice.

A recent study provided evidence that most nurses provide care in accordance with what they learned in nursing school and rarely used journal articles, research reports, and hospital libraries for reference (Pravikoff, Tanner, & Pierce, 2005). That finding, combined with the fact that the average nurse is more than 40 years of age, makes it apparent that many nurses' knowledge is probably outdated. Practice based on such knowledge does not translate into quality patient care or health outcomes. Evidence-based practice provides a critical strategy to ensure that care is up to date and that it reflects the latest research evidence.

Tips for Success

Why bother with EBP? It allows nurses to implement the most up-to-date, research-tested, and high-quality patient care.

Why is EBP important to nursing practice?

- It results in better patient outcomes

- It contributes to the science of nursing

- It keeps practice current and relevant

- It increases confidence in decision-making

- Policies and procedures are current and include the latest research, thus supporting JCAHO-readiness

- Integration of EBP into nursing practice is essential for high-quality patient care and achievement of ANCC Magnet Recognition Program® (MRP) designation

Often, nurses feel that they are using "evidence" to guide practice, but their sources of evidence are not research-based. In a study conducted by Thompson, et al., (2003), nurses reported that the most helpful knowledge source was experience or advice from colleagues or patients. Of concern were reports that up-to-date electronic resources that included evidence-based materials were not useful to nurses in clinical practice. This barrier contributes to significant gaps in clinicians applying research findings to practice and dissemination of innovations. The failure to use evidence results in care that is of lower quality, less effective, and more expensive (Berwick, 2003).

Evidence-based practice can be easier for nurses to use if they refer to already-developed evidence-based or clinical practice guidelines. Numerous expert groups have already undertaken systematic efforts to develop guidelines to help both healthcare providers and patients make informed decisions about care interventions. Guideline developers use a systematic approach to critique the existing research, rate the strength of the evidence, and establish practice guidelines. The overall goal of these types of efforts focuses on guiding practice and minimizing the variability in care.

For example in 2002, the Centers for Disease Control and Prevention published *Guideline for Hand Hygiene in Health-Care Settings*, which provides healthcare workers with a review of data regarding hand-washing and hand antisepsis in healthcare environments. Furthermore, it makes recommendations to improve hand-hygiene practices and reduce transmission of pathogenic microorganisms to both patients and healthcare personnel. See Chapter 3 for further discussion of accessing clinical practice guidelines.

What are the barriers to implementing evidence-based practice?

The barriers that prevent nurses from using research in everyday practice have been cited in numerous studies, and some common findings have emerged (Clifford & Murray, 2001; Funk, Champagne, Wiese, & Tornquist, 1991; Newhouse, Dearholt, Poe, Pugh, & White, 2005; Pravikoff, et al., 2005). Nurses often report the following:

- Lack of value for research in practice
- Difficulty in changing practice
- Lack of administrative support
- Lack of knowledgeable mentors
- Insufficient time to conduct research
- Lack of education about the research process
- Lack of awareness about research or evidence-based practice
- Research reports/articles not readily available
- Difficulty accessing research reports and articles
- No time on the job to read research
- Complexity of research reports

- Lack of knowledge about EBP and critique of articles
- Feeling overwhelmed by the process

Despite these barriers, nurses are engaging in EBP and making a difference in patient outcomes. Furthermore, barriers can be overcome through organizational efforts focused on integrating research in practice and using strategies such as journal clubs, nursing grand rounds, and having research articles available for review (Fink, Thompson, & Bonnes, 2005). Case studies presented in Chapter 8 showcase the integration of EBP into everyday nursing practice.

Is your organization ready for the challenge? Are you ready for the challenge? Do the supports and resources exist in your environment? To be successful with evidence-based practice, one needs to be willing to challenge one's own assumptions and be willing to work with others to improve care processes and patient outcomes. Evidence-based practice takes resources, work, time, and effort, but the outcomes make them worthwhile. Every patient deserves care that is based on the best scientific knowledge and that ensures high-quality, cost-effective care.

Practice exercises

1. Log on to the Cochrane Collaboration Web site at *www.cochrane.org*. Find the topic list and read some reviews. Did you find information on this site useful to your practice setting? Why or why not?

2. Develop a list of the resources you need to participate in evidence-based practice. Identify resources that exist in your organization. Consider ways of accessing resources that do not currently exist in your clinical setting. Create an action plan for getting involved in evidence-based practice, and include a time frame and economic resources. Identify potential collaborators for your efforts related to evidence-based practice.

3. Visit *www.hospitalcompare.hhs.gov* and compare the performance of hospitals in your town/city, region, or state. Ask your colleagues whether they know about public reporting. Find out more about what your organization is doing to address acute myocardial infarction care, heart failure care, and pneumonia care. Learn more about multidisciplinary evidence-based projects in your organization.

4. Do a Web search on "evidence-based nursing." Review various Web resources to identify the most helpful Web sites. Visit a medical or public library and learn more about evidence-based resources that patients might access to inform themselves about their health condition or related interventions.

References

Berwick, D. M. (2003). Disseminating innovations in health care. *The Journal of the American Medical Association, 289* (15), 1969–1975.

Centers for Disease Control and Prevention. (2002). Guideline for Hand Hygiene in Health-Care Settings. Retrieved January 3, 2006, from www.cdc.gov/mmwr/preview/mmwrhtml/rr5116a1.htm.

Clifford, C., & Murray, S. (2001). Pre- and post-test evaluation of a project to facilitate research development in practice in a hospital setting. *Journal of Advanced Nursing, 36* (5), 685–695.

Fink, R., Thompson, C. J., & Bonnes, D. (2005). Overcoming barriers and promoting the use of research in practice. *Journal of Nursing Administration, 35* (3), 121–129.

Funk, S. G., Champagne, M.T., Wiese, R.A., & Tornquist, E.M. (1991). Barriers to using research findings in practice: the clinician's perspective. *Applied Nursing Research, 4* (2), 90–95.

Madsen, D., Sebolt, T., Cullen, L., Folkedahl, B., Mueller, T., Richardson, C., et al. (2005). Listening to bowel sounds: An evidence-based practice project. *American Journal of Nursing, 105* (12), 40–49.

Nelson, E. C., Batalden, P.B., Huber, T.P., Mohr, J.R., Godfrey, M.M., Headrick, L.A., et al. (2002). Microsystems in health care: Part 1. Learning from high-performing front-line clinical units. *The Joint Commission Journal on Quality Improvement, 28* (9), 472–493.

Newhouse, R., Dearholt, S., Poe, S., Pugh, L.C., & White, K.M. (2005). Evidence-based practice: a practical approach to implementation. *Journal of Nursing Administration, 35* (1), 35–40.

Pravikoff, D. S., Tanner, A.B., & Pierce, S.T. (2005). Readiness of U. S. nurses for evidence-based practice. *American Journal of Nursing, 105* (9), 40–51.

Sackett, D. L., Rosenberg, W.M.C., Gray, M.J.A., Hayes, R.B., & Richardson W.S. (1996). Evidence-based medicine: What it is and what it isn't. *British Medical Journal, 312,* 71–72.

Thompson, C., McCaughan, D., Cullum, N., Sheldon, T.A., Munhall, A., & Thompson, D.R. (2001). Research information in nurses' clinical decision-making: What is useful. *Journal of Advanced Nursing, 36* (3), 376–388.

Burns, N., & Grove, S. (2001.) *The Practice of Nursing Research: Conduct, Critique, and Utilization.* (4th ed.) Philadelphia: W.B. Saunders Company.

Polit, D.F. & Beck, C.T. (2003.) *Nursing Research: Principles and Methods.* (7th ed.) Philadelphia: Lippincott Williams & Wilkins.

Polit, D.F. & Beck, C.T. (2003). *Study Guide to Accompany Nursing Research: Principles and Methods.* (7th ed.) Philadelphia: Lippincott Williams & Wilkins.

Integration of evidence-based practice

Learning objectives

After reading this chapter, the participant should be able to
- identify strategies to establish a culture for inquiry and EBP
- discuss approaches for nurses to participate in EBP and research

First steps to evidence-based practice

Evidence-based practice does not just happen because it is the right thing to do or because a nursing organization wants to seek designation from the American Nurses Credentialing Center's Magnet Recognition Program®. Evidence-based practice is not the latest buzzword or trend in healthcare; instead, it must be highly valued as the right way to provide healthcare and leadership while establishing a framework for safety and quality. For a nursing organization to be successful in evidence-based practice efforts, numerous essential supports and resources must be readily available.

The leadership and vision of the chief nurse executive (CNE) are integral components to creating, advancing, and sustaining a practice environment grounded in evidence-based practice. As discussed in Chapter 1, although the terms "nursing research" and "evidence-based practice" are often used interchangeably, they are not the same. Nursing research has been described as a systematic inquiry that uses defined, scientific methods to answer questions or solve problems, whereas evidence-based practice uses research findings to guide clinical decisions, actions, interventions, and policies.

The CNE provides leadership for the professional practice nursing environment within a healthcare organization. To create that environment, he or she establishes goals and objectives and allocates resources for the nursing organization in conjunction with the nursing leadership team. The CNE must believe in and provide support for the idea that evidence-based management and nursing practice serve as an essential framework for high-quality patient care. Without such a commitment to evidence-based practice by each member of the nursing leadership team, efforts to achieve success may be somewhat limited by that lack of support.

Creating a culture of evidence-based practice

For nurses to value and recognize the relevance and importance of evidence-based practice, they need ongoing support from the CNE and the nursing leadership team. The leadership team must encourage nurses' efforts to question existing practice, have access to library resources and research experts, and provide time for nurses to work on evidence-based projects. Most importantly, the nursing leadership team must value clinical inquiry, scholarship, and questioning of the status quo. Staff nurses must be empowered to use evidence to improve their practice and must have the resources to accomplish goals related to improving the quality and safety of nursing care.

Nurses' lack of experience or expertise in the evidence-based practice process is a common and significant barrier for nurse clinicians and leaders who want to encourage EBP at their facilities. In this instance, numerous strategies already exist that nursing leaders can consider in supporting evidence-based practice efforts. For example, the CNE may schedule a series of workshops for nurses interested in learning more about research and evidence-based practice. Participants could be interested staff nurses, nurse educators, clinical nurse specialists, and advanced practice nurses. Another possible strategy is to collaborate with or employ a nurse researcher who can support the formation of a research or evidence-based practice council, work with staff nurses on evidence-based projects, and provide education to and mentor interested individuals or groups.

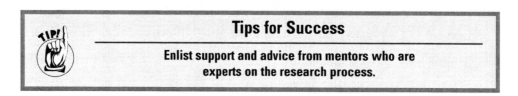

Tips for Success

Enlist support and advice from mentors who are experts on the research process.

Many healthcare organizations develop a collaborative relationship with a local school of nursing and, through a joint appointment arrangement, acquire the part-time services of a nurse researcher. Such agreements often benefit both the school of nursing and the healthcare organization and can result in synergies between research efforts of nursing students and staff members. If an organization

Tips for Success

Hold workshops for anyone
interested in learning more about EBP.

cannot afford the services of a nurse researcher, other individuals who may serve as mentors in the research process may include masters-prepared advanced practice nurses (APN) or clinical nurse specialists (CNS). Remember, one of the most critical resources in the research process is support from mentors who are expert in the process. If an organization lacks these resources, finding opportunities to collaborate with organizations that do have and can share the needed research expertise becomes another viable strategy.

Most importantly, the strategies used should be a fit with the culture and readiness of the nursing organization. For example, the CNE may not initially have the financial resources to employ a nurse researcher, so a first step to evidence-based practice might be to require the use of at least two research articles in the development or revision of nursing policies and procedures. This requirement will help nurses learn about the library resources available at their institution and begin to learn how to read the research. In another setting, it might be appropriate to hire a nurse researcher to support the ongoing evidence-based practice efforts of existing staff nurses. In yet another, the staff nurses may be ready for a nurse researcher to come in and develop and implement a research program. The variation between organizations means that the nursing leadership team must assess the organization's readiness for evidence-based practice and match the resources to the clinical environment before embarking on the journey.

Time and resources to allow EBP to flourish

Creating a culture where evidence-based practice can flourish requires resources such as subscriptions to electronic journals and databases, access to computers and the Internet, and release time for staff nurses to work on projects and to serve on evidence-based councils. There is no such thing as research on a shoestring budget, and although the hard work of dedicated professionals can bring high-quality results, it does take time and resources. Evidence-based projects rarely occur without the combined expertise of a group of clinicians who can readily access the literature and who have the time to work on a specific project. Therefore, some first steps to developing an evidence-based culture can be assessing the accessibility of electronic resources and computers and developing a plan so that those resources are available to staff nurses.

Tips for Success

Make sure you have ready access to computers and other electronic resources.

Also consider providing nurses with education about the importance of evidence-based practice and how it fits into their daily work. This education includes helping nurses learn how to search the literature, access resources, critique published research articles, develop and implement a research protocol, and disseminate the results of a research or evidence-based project. Encourage nurses to attend seminars or conferences that include research reports to help them learn more about research. Some organizations offer continuing education programs on evidence-based practice or collaborate with a local school of nursing to offer an on-site research course for academic credit. Again, the specific educational offerings must fit the culture of the organization and the needs and readiness of the staff members. There is limited use in trying to get nurses involved in research or evidence-based practice if they are working mandatory overtime or if limited resources or support exist for professional development or practice.

Tips for Success

Allow staff nurses time away from the bedside to undertake research.

Creating a forum for discussion

EBP or nursing research council

Forming an EBP or nursing research council offers a forum where nurses can begin discussing areas of interest, coordinating journal clubs, and receiving education about evidence-based practice and nursing research. The membership of the committee should include associate, baccalaureate, and masters prepared nurses and represent clinical departments throughout the organization. Members of the nursing research or evidence-based council will energize each other and share their knowledge as they learn how to read and critique research articles or proposals, initiate EBP projects, and possibly write or implement a research proposal.

Members of this group can become champions for evidence-based practice. The opportunity to develop their expertise and skills provides a foundation for research and evidence-based efforts throughout the nursing organization. A nursing research or evidence-based practice council can focus on activities of concern to all practice settings or develop specialty or topic subgroups to work on specific efforts. Featuring the work of the council through newsletters, posters, nursing grand rounds, and continuing education offerings within one's own organization helps disseminate information while highlighting the importance of evidence-based practice. EBP/nursing research councils are discussed in detail in Chapter 4.

Nursing practice committees and other forums

The research or evidence-based council cannot be the only forum in which the importance of research and evidence-based practice is discussed. In every situation where nurses come together to discuss practice or administrative issues or problems, someone needs to ask the question, "What research exists on this topic?" Opportunities to use evidence-based practice exist on nursing practice committees whether they are organization-wide or unit-based, as well as in every clinical and administrative situation. Do not underestimate the importance of answering questions with evidence.

For example, the value analysis or product committee might consider adopting a new device. In this instance, it would be important to ask the question, "What evidence exists that this is a better product?" It would be foolish to purchase new equipment just because it is available. Likewise, if the administrative team is considering scheduling changes, the group should examine the latest evidence on work hours and their relationship to medical errors and patient safety. An infection control committee might make a recommendation to change an infection control procedure, and again the question should be asked, "What is the evidence for this change?" In this way, members of the team make every decision using the latest information and an evidence-based problem-solving approach.

The benefits of using an evidence-based approach include reviewing the most recently published research findings and not relying on one's personal expertise or experience. In this way, best practices can be developed using a knowledge-based rather than an opinion-based approach, and thus evidence-based practices emerge as the organizational standard and expectation. Examining the evidence provides an essential framework for problem solving and making well-informed decisions.

If only a few people are involved in implementing evidence-based practice, it will quickly become the latest fad and not the framework for clinical practice and management. Regardless of the situation, all clinicians and administrative personnel need to feel free to ask the difficult questions, "Why do we do it this way?" or "Does this practice make sense?" Then everyone needs to feel comfortable in accessing the resources that can help answer these difficult questions.

Identifying areas of concern

Staff nurses must be active participants in identifying clinical questions that can be solved or addressed with evidence-based practice. Although faculty members, APNs, CNSs, nursing leaders, and researchers can facilitate the process, they should not dictate the topics to be investigated. Staff nurses need to identify and prioritize the topics of interest to help ensure excitement, acceptance, and application at the bedside. Initially, topics should be broad and do not have to be written as "a focused EBP or research question."

The EBP/nursing research council can serve as the starting point for dialogue. One approach to help identify topic areas is to ask nurses to

- identify nursing activities that they believe are a waste of time or that seem futile
- describe a nursing practice based on myth or tradition
- discuss a gap between practice and a recently published research article
- question a specific nursing technique or procedure
- describe a nursing intervention that results in more harm or waste than benefit
- identify a patient problem that is costly or otherwise wastes resources

Examples of broad topics include the following:

- Family presence during CPR
- Family visitation in the post-anesthesia unit
- Verifying placement of nasogastric tubes
- Pain assessment and management
- Prevention of ventilator-associated pneumonia
- Eliminating bloodstream infections related to central lines
- Pet visitation
- Best practices for oral care for intubated patients
- Best practices for tube feedings
- Safe administration of medications
- Work environment and decision-making
- Fatigue and medical error
- Reconciling medications

Regardless of whether they are in clinical or administrative roles, nurses want to solve real-life problems. Making nursing research interesting and pertinent to nurses and their current practice environment helps ensure their involvement in and commitment to the process.

Creating internal expertise

Once administrative support is in place and nurses become excited about undertaking projects and changing practice, start developing expertise about evidence-based practice. Initially, nurses could learn to navigate electronic databases and could investigate journals that are available in either print or electronic copy in their organization. If no journals or databases are available, the same outcome can be obtained by visiting a local hospital that is doing EBP and seeing what journals and electronic databases they have in place. If the organization has partnered with a local college of nursing, have nursing staff members schedule an appointment with the reference librarian to learn how to access the available resources. If there is no dedicated medical or nursing library readily available, the local community library may have resources, such as PubMed, that can help you begin to build evidence-based practice resources.

Tips for Success

Online editions of journals provide quick and easy access to research when first starting EBP.

The EBP/nursing research council can organize a list of available journals and databases and start coordinating educational sessions. One approach that works with nurses who are novices with research is to focus the initial EBP/nursing research council meetings on education. Emphasizing education rather than on identifying research questions, selecting an EBP model, reviewing protocol, or designing studies allows staff nurses the time to develop their skills. This strategy helps ease interested staff nurses into a contributory role as they participate in the work of the group and build their skill levels. Initial topics for the educational sessions could include the following:

- How do I undertake a literature search?
- What is evidence-based practice?
- Is evidence-based practice for me?
- Why is evidence-based practice important to my patients and to our organization?

- How do we find time for evidence-based practice?
- How do I get started?
- What resources do I need?
- What resources are available?

One of the biggest challenges nurses face is learning how to search the literature. Having a librarian or educator come to the meeting with a laptop computer and do a "real-time" search will build nurses' confidence in the process of searching electronic resources. As the group continues to develop knowledge and awareness, more advanced topics can be added, such as

- levels of evidence
- critique of qualitative research articles
- critique of quantitative research articles
- critique of research proposals
- protection of human subjects
- ethical issues in nursing research
- reliability and validity
- overview of models of EBP
- formulating an EBP or research question
- synthesizing the literature
- developing a clinical practice guideline

Three major barriers often prevent research from being translated into practice: difficulty finding research articles, uncertainty about evaluating research, and difficulty with interpreting findings. Participation in journal clubs enhances nurses' confidence in all of these areas and prepares nurses for critiquing research, which is an essential component of evidence-based practice. When conducting journal clubs, a group of nurses meets regularly to discuss and critique articles from nursing research journals. Articles are evaluated for scientific integrity and relevance to nursing practice.

The journal club format allows members of the nursing staff to become active participants in EBP. It serves as a way to bridge research and practice, and thereby fosters the application of research findings into the practice setting. The traditional approach to a journal club is for nurses to meet as a group for about an hour to critique an article. However, practice realities can make this difficult to accomplish on a routine basis in some clinical settings, so after the group is comfortable reading, discussing, and evaluating articles, consider alternative approaches, such as electronic resources for online journal clubs. See Chapter 5 for more on journal clubs.

Another strategy that helps nurses develop expertise in evidence-based practice is to have them develop policies and procedures. Encouraging nurses to develop or update policies and procedures using the latest research findings helps introduce them to the research literature. Working together in small groups, nurses can encourage and support each other in interpreting the findings from various research studies and developing evidence-based practice.

Once nurses have become comfortable reading and discussing articles, they are ready to start doing formal critiques of the nursing literature. Guidelines for critique of research articles will be presented in Chapter 5. Additional guidelines are available in nursing research textbooks or can be developed for your organizational needs by an advance practice nurse or research consultant. For example, before using nursing research articles for policies and procedures or to validate or change practice, one must ask the following questions:

- Where was the study conducted? What was the setting (e.g., academic medical center, community hospital, rural hospital, or long-term care facility)?

- Who was in the study population? Were study participants similar to patients cared for in this organization?

- How does the study contribute to the body of nursing knowledge? Do the study findings make sense?

- What are the implications for nursing practice/education/research?

- What additional questions does the study raise?

- Does the empirical evidence presented in this article support a change in practice?

- What resources would be required to implement the change?

- Would the benefits of this practice change or outweigh the risks to patients?

- What will be the outcome of this practice change on nurses, patients, or the organization?

- How will the practice change be evaluated?

Another way to develop nurses' skills is to encourage nurses to be active participants in any evidence-based practice efforts being conducted by multidisciplinary teams. For example, the surgeons in a particular hospital might conduct an improvement effort related to preventing surgical-site infections. Including nurses in this effort provides them with an opportunity to learn while they contribute to the effort. Examining problems from a multidisciplinary perspective also benefits patients and their families by ensuring best practices.

Getting started in research and evidence-based practice begins by identifying problems and prioritizing projects. Identifying situations that result in negative or unexpected clinical outcomes or by examining hunches made from clinical observations is another important way to develop research questions. Perhaps one of the most important ways to become successful in research is to ask questions that are of interest and importance. More important than knowledge about research, then, is asking questions that have true clinical meaning and pursuing them with great passion (Beyea, 2000).

Putting research into action

When deciding to make evidence-based practice changes, evaluate the outcomes of any changes. Never assume that changes in clinical practice will have the anticipated outcomes. Therefore, pilot-test the changes on one or two clinical units to help detect unexpected outcomes and to understand any implementation-related problems. Based on the findings from the pilot units, you can decide to move forward with the practice change in all of the applicable units or to modify or reject the change.

Even if the implementation is successful, the project is not complete. Any evidence-based project requires clinicians to monitor the findings in an ongoing fashion. New knowledge or information can be developed and will need to be integrated into the practice change. Evidence-based projects are never complete—they require the continuous efforts of dedicated professionals who are willing to question their practice and continually find ways to improve patient outcomes.

Tips for Success

Anticipate that changes to clinical practice may present challenges and may not have the anticipated outcome.

Share the knowledge

Disseminating and publicizing the results of EBP projects supports the culture of evidence-based practice. It serves a critical role in advancing nursing and increasing staff nurse involvement in nursing scholarship efforts. Findings from the EBP/nursing research council or unit-based efforts can be displayed on posters in the cafeteria or other areas. Information about projects also can be described in the healthcare organization's or nursing department's newsletters, whether printed or electronic. Some hospitals have a nursing EBP project day during which certain projects are presented as papers and others are offered in a poster format. Additional dissemination efforts can include poster presentations at local, regional, or national conferences. Staff nurses also should be encouraged to develop articles for nursing journals. Helping staff nurses understand the importance of contributing to nursing science in this way helps them understand the importance of their work and its value to patients and the larger nursing community.

Practice exercises

1. Identify the types of administrative and research supports in place for EBP that exist within your organization.

2. Explore how registered nurses can be paid or given release time to attend EBP meetings or do EBP projects.

3. Explore possible linkages with a local school of nursing and determine the availability of research mentors.

4. Schedule an appointment with your hospital librarian to see what journals and databases are available, and learn how to do a review of the literature. If you do not have a library, check with a local school of nursing or another hospital in your area to find out what journals and databases are available.

5. Ask patients what resources they use when they want to learn more about their health. Examine pertinent evidence-based guidelines for health screenings and determine whether your healthcare provider recommended laboratory and diagnostic testing in accordance with evidence-based recommendations.

References

Beyea, S. C. (2000). "Getting started in nursing research and tips for success." *AORN Journal, 72* (6), 1061–1062.

Further reading

Brown, Sarah Jo. (1999). *Knowledge for Health Care Practice: A Guide to Using Research Evidence*. Philadelphia: W.B. Saunders Company.

Fain, James A. (2003). *Reading, Understanding and Applying Nursing Research: A Text and Workbook*. (2nd ed.) Philadelphia: F. A. Davis Company.

Melnyk, B.M., & Fineout-Overholt, E. (2004). *Evidence-Based Practice in Nursing and Healthcare: A Guide to Best Practice*. Philadelphia: Lippincott Williams & Wilkins.

Sams, L., Penn, B.K., & Facteau, L. (2004). The challenge of using evidence-based practice. *Journal of Nursing Administration, 34* (9), 407–414.

Scott-Findlay, S. & Golden-Biddle, K. (2005). Understanding how organizational culture shapes research use. *Journal of Nursing Administration, 35* (7–8), 359–365.

Accessing and appraising resources

Learning objectives

After reading this chapter, the participant should be able to
- describe approaches to finding pertinent and reliable literature and research
- discuss various approaches to appraising the strength of the evidence

Resources are widely available

When many current nurses were students, going to the library was an adventure in books and other printed materials. Doing research in the library was a somewhat formidable task: First, you had to find the indexes to the literature, which were thick and presented in multiple volumes, and then explore for journal articles in another part of the library, taking notes on index cards (especially in the days before readily accessible copiers), and finally waiting for weeks for an interlibrary loan request. The library served as a place where one went to do research, and more often than not, it was far removed from clinical environments.

Today, many of these same resources are accessible without a trip to the library and can be accessed at the point of care with the click of a computer mouse. Many journals, books, and indexes are available in an electronic format, and busy clinicians can effortlessly print a selected article within moments. An interlibrary loan can be achieved by making an electronic request.

Thus, for many clinicians, the trip to the library is a virtual journey that can be accomplished without ever moving away from the computer. Other clinicians have varying degrees of access to these electronic resources or may not work in an agency that provides any electronic resources. This chapter will address searching and accessing the literature and research with a focus on electronic resources, which are available in many settings. If these electronic resources are not readily available, this chapter will provide guidance on how to access these resources at home or at a local community library.

Searching for evidence

Electronic resources are the primary ways to search the literature and are available in both fee-for-service and free modalities. Searching most electronic resources requires access to the Internet and, thus, a computer, so the first thing a nurse needs is access to the Internet. Nurses often can access the Internet without paying additional fees by using their local public library or using resources at work. A nurse also could establish a relationship with an Internet Service Provider (ISP) and pay any associated fees.

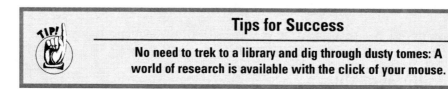

Tips for Success

No need to trek to a library and dig through dusty tomes: A world of research is available with the click of your mouse.

Internet access allows nurses to use electronic indexes, including those provided by the National Library of Medicine. Many hospitals and schools of nursing also purchase or subscribe to a variety software developed to help clinicians and others search the Cumulative Index for Nursing and Allied Health (CINAHL) (*www.cinahl.com*), Medline (*www.nlm.nih.gov*), or other health-related indexes. Another popular resource for searching the literature is PubMed (*www.pubmed.gov*), which is the National Library of Medicine's free, Web-based format of Medline.

Topic-specific indexes

Numerous topic-specific electronic indexes are available, and depending upon the type of search you are doing, it may be helpful to explore beyond the traditional nursing and medical reference indexes. Other indexes address social sciences, consumer health, books, audiovisual materials, healthcare delivery, and education. Information about these various indexes is available from the local community or college library. Often it is helpful to search fields that are related to nursing when conducting an EBP project, as research derived in another field may be relevant and may guide practice in a helpful manner.

Tips for Success

Clearly define your search to avoid being buried
under an avalanche of sources.

Search engines

Another popular, but less scientific, approach to searching for information is using a search engine. For example, entering the terms "breast cancer" and "nursing" in a popular search engine results in hundreds of links to information and journal articles related to the topic. PubMed, in contrast, only identifies journal articles. In using PubMed, one can limit a search to research articles or to a certain timeframe, author, or various other defined limits. Such Web searches can help identify other evidence-based projects and linkages when a literature search does not yield pertinent resources. For example, little has been written or published about falls-risk assessment in children. A recent Web search helped a clinical nurse specialist in her efforts to identify risk assessments used in other clinical settings and connect with individuals who have been working on this topic.

To conduct a search, first identify a topic of interest and then start the search. In some instances, you may need to narrow or broaden the topic. For example, perhaps the unit-based nursing practice committee wants to reduce the incidence of infections related to urinary catheters. If you enter the search term "catheters" in PubMed, it identifies approximately 143,000 articles. Obviously, this search must be narrowed. On the next try, "urinary catheters" is entered as the search term, and PubMed identifies approximately 14,000 articles. If you further limit the search by using "urinary catheter and infection," you get approximately 4,000 articles. Obviously, that would still be too many articles to read and review, so narrowing the topic further is most important. Further limiting the search to randomized control studies, English-language only, and nursing journal articles results in a much shorter list of only four pertinent articles. Changing the limits to include review articles in Medline results in a reference list of 104 articles, which might be a good starting point for this particular evidence-based project.

Electronic indexes

Electronic indexes provide users with many options for narrowing or broadening the topic and helping identify the relevant literature and resources. Another helpful limit that many biomedical libraries offer is an interface between certain indexes and the listing of existing library resources. In this way, the search yields information about whether the resource is available in a specific library. Some paper-based indexes continue to be available, but most libraries have chosen electronic options, so learning about electronic indexes helps anyone doing evidence-based projects.

Once the search has been conducted, review the list and determine which articles should be reviewed. Most available electronic resources provide citation information such as the author(s) name(s), the title, publication information, and search times. Many biomedical libraries provide a link within the search results that allows end-users to access or order the electronic version of the item or indicates whether a print copy is available locally. In this way, you can get a copy of the article by just a few clicks of the mouse. Results from a search can be printed for future review, saved as an electronic file, or imported to another software program for manuscript development. Another helpful feature of most indexes is that a reference list can be imported into a bibliographic database, which can be a big help in managing reference lists. To learn more about bibliographic managers, visit the following Web pages:

- Albert Einstein College of Medicine (*http://library.aecom.yu.edu/resources/bms/bmsfaq.htm*)

- Gerstein Science Information Centre (*www.library.utoronto.ca/gerstein/subjectguides/personalbib.html*)

Electronic resources

A few of the many other helpful Internet resources for evidence-based practice include the National Library of Medicine, the Cochrane Library of Databases, the National Guideline Clearinghouse, the Joanna Briggs Institute, and Netting the Evidence, among others.

Learning more about each of these resources serves as an important first step to evidence-based practice. The materials available on each of these sites provide a beginning understanding of many of the resources clinicians can access when undertaking evidence-based projects. Many of these Web sites provide links to resources that also may be helpful.

National Library of Medicine

The National Library of Medicine serves as a key resource for many databases in addition to those on Medline, and those databases may be pertinent to various evidence-based projects. Those services and catalogues are described in detail on the NLM's Webpage (*www.nlm.nih.gov*). Resources available through the NLM include MedlinePlus, ClinicalTrials.gov, NIHSeniorHealth, ToxTown, Household Products, Genetics Home Reference (GHR), and AIDSinfo. Each of these databases includes topic-specific information that may relate to focused evidence-based projects. For example, perhaps the effort relates to the care of AIDS patients. A key resource in that effort would be AIDSinfo, which offers current information on clinical trials for AIDS patients and federally approved HIV treatment and prevention guidelines.

Cochrane Library

The abstracts of the various reviews are available free of charge on the Cochrane Library Web site (*www.cochrane.org/reviews/clibintro.htm*) and provide a valuable source of healthcare information. In some instances, plain-language summaries also are provided using a minimum of technical terms. Many biomedical libraries give users access to some or all of these databases. A popular resource is the Cochrane Database of Systematic Reviews, which provides systematic reviews that reflect the best available information about healthcare interventions and their effectiveness. Expert teams complete comprehensive literature and research reviews, evaluate the research, and present integrated summaries of the best evidence. These reviews are updated on a regular basis and incorporate new research findings when they become available.

The Cochrane Library includes the following databases:

- Cochrane Database of Systematic Reviews
- Database of Abstracts of Reviews of Effects
- Cochrane Controlled Trials Register
- Cochrane Methodology Register
- NHS Economic Evaluation Database
- Health Technology Assessment Database
- Cochrane Database of Methodology Reviews (CDMR)

National Guideline Clearinghouse

The National Guideline Clearinghouse (NGC) (*www.ngc.gov*) provides a virtual resource for evidence-based protocols. Currently, the NGC database contains more than 1,700 guidelines. This public resource is an initiative of the Agency for Healthcare Research and Quality (AHRQ). Such protocols or guidelines are developed by teams of experts who have reviewed and synthesized the literature, and rated the strength of the research findings, thus providing clinicians and patients guidance about best practices for a particular condition. This searchable Web site allows users to search by disease or condition, measures or tools, and the developing organization; it also includes review guidelines that are in progress or those that have been archived. On this Web site, a search using the terms "urinary catheters and infection," results in 11 guidelines that may be pertinent to the effort.

Joanna Briggs Institute

The Joanna Briggs Institute (*www.joannabriggs.edu.au*) supports a "collaborative approach to the evaluation of evidence from a diverse range of sources, including experience, expertise, and all forms of vigorous research" and the implementation of the best available evidence. The Institute brings together practice-oriented research activities to improve effectiveness, processes, and outcomes. Included among some of its activities are

- conducting systematic reviews of the research
- collaborating with expert researchers and clinicians to develop best practices
- offering courses in evidence-based nursing
- primary research when indicated by the findings of the systematic review
- promoting cost-effective, evidence-based nursing
- planning and organizing research colloquia

The Web page provides comprehensive nursing resources and opportunities to collaborate with others interested in similar efforts and projects.

Netting the Evidence

Another helpful resource is "Netting the Evidence" (*www.shef.ac.uk/scharr/ir/netting*). This Web site provides a searchable database for finding evidence for practice. Users can find quick links to various Internet resources that can answer statistical questions, guide bedside diagnosis, access evidence-based practice guideline databases, and explore a wide variety of other evidence-based resources. This searchable database is intended to facilitate evidence-based healthcare by providing support and access to useful learning resources, including an evidence-based virtual library, software, and journals.

Centre for Evidence-based Medicine University Health Network

Some electronic resources may be helpful to evidence-based councils in their efforts to develop knowledge and skills when embarking on the evidence-based practice journey. For example, the Centre for Evidence-based Medicine University Health Network (*www.library.utoronto.ca/medicine/ebm/*) provides numerous resources to help develop, disseminate, and evaluate resources for teaching and practicing evidence-based medicine. The headings on their home page include an introduction to evidence-based medicine, syllabi for practicing evidence-based medicine, evidence resources, a glossary, and many other resources.

Centre for Health Evidence

Another Web site that might be helpful in developing evidence-based practice expertise is the Canadian Centre for Health Evidence (*www.cche.net*). This resource intends to help patients, clinicians, and policymakers by providing resources and helping people acquire, appraise, and use knowledge and develop an understanding of how the information is used. One of the many helpful resources on this site includes numerous articles on evidence-based practice that are available in a downloadable format. These articles would be especially helpful to any organization that lacks electronic library resources.

Registered Nurses Association of Ontario

One particularly helpful resource for nurses is provided by the Registered Nurses Association of Ontario (*www.rnao.org/bestpractices/about/bestPractice_overview.asp*). Their Nursing Best Practice Guidelines (NBPG) program supports Ontario nurses by providing them with best practice guidelines for patient care. The program includes cycles of five phases: planning, development, pilot implementation, evaluation, and dissemination/uptake. At present, this program focuses on gerontology, primary healthcare, home healthcare, mental healthcare, and emergency care. They have also developed 29 guidelines, a toolkit for implementing the guidelines, and an educator's resource.

Other Web resources

Numerous other nursing-specific, evidence-based Web resources have been developed, including the following:

- University of Minnesota (*http://evidence.ahc.umn.edu/ebn.htm*)

- Centre for Evidence Based Nursing (*www.york.ac.uk/healthsciences/centres/evidence/cebn.htm*)

- McGill University Health Centre's Research and Clinical Resources of Evidence Based Nursing (*www.muhc-ebn.mcgill.ca*)

- University of North Carolina Health Science Library (*www.hsl.unc.edu/Services/Tutorials/EBN/index.htm*)

• Academic Center for Evidence-Based Nursing (*www.acestar.uthscsa.edu*)

This list is not a comprehensive listing resource, but it provides a beginning point for individuals and groups that want to learn more. Using the term "evidence-based practice" can result in millions of possible links when conducting a simple Web search. The links provided here narrow that initial search and offer some opportunities to learn the basics while exploring additional Web sites.

Evaluating evidence

Nurses need to always evaluate evidence, regardless of the sources. Indeed, even the spoken word should be assessed for its reliability and validity. Therefore, the first rule of evaluating evidence includes determining the source of the information, when it was developed, how it was developed, and whether it fits the current clinical environment and situation. For example, knowledge derived from mercury thermometers may be outdated in light of a current practice environment that uses only electronic thermometers.

Statements that start with "research shows that this is true" should always be questioned, and nurses should consistently ask for the primary source. That means finding, reading, and examining the evidence. Nurses are accustomed to learning from experts such as their faculty, colleagues, or physicians, so questioning the evidence may be a somewhat new experience. These experts and other authorities have often served as the opinion leaders within our educational and practice settings, but by challenging the evidence, each nurse can become better informed.

Tips for Success

Avoid taking Web resources at face value. Look for the primary source of the evidence and evaluate how conclusions were reached.

Evaluate Web sites

When examining Web pages and the content within these resources, conduct a systematic evaluation of the information's worth. A simple mnemonic that can be used to evaluate Web sites is, "Are you PLEASED with this site?"

• Purpose of the site—Determine whether the purpose is clearly explained and whether it fits the content on the site.

- Links—Determine whether the links are current and whether they link to reputable sources.

- Editorial—Determine whether the content is up to date and correct.

- Author—Identify the author and his or her credentials for providing the presented information.

- Site—When reviewing the site, evaluate its ease of use and how the content is presented.

- Ethical—Consider whether contact information for the author is readily available and whether appropriate disclosures about the content are provided.

- Dates—Ask when the information was posted and whether the Web site has been recently reviewed and updated (Nicoll & Beyea, 2000).

This approach is one way to evaluate Web content. Multiple resources exist to evaluate medical information on the Internet. Some Web sites that might be helpful in guiding the evaluation process include the following:

- Johns Hopkins Library (*www.library.jhu.edu/researchhelp/general/evaluating*)

- University of California Berkeley Library (*www.lib.berkeley.edu/TeachingLib/Guides /Internet/Evaluate.html*)

- Cornell Library (*www.library.cornell.edu/olinuris/ref/research/skill26.htm*)

Numerous other resources exist to help clinicians learn to evaluate Web resources, but these sites are a place to get started in efforts to learn about the process.

DISCERN tool

A resource that all health consumers should know about is the DISCERN Instrument (*www.discern. org.uk*). This standardized instrument helps evaluate the reliability and quality of consumer health information. It consists of 15 key questions, plus an overall quality rating. By using the DISCERN Instrument, consumers can become involved in a shared decision-making process about their treatment choices. Using this instrument, consumers can determine whether the information they are reviewing is based on good evidence and whether it should be used or discarded.

FIGURE 3.1

The DISCERN Instrument

SECTION 1
Is the publication reliable?

1. Are the aims clear?

Rating this question

No		Partially		Yes
1	2	3	4	5

HINT: Look for a clear indication at the beginning of the publication of:
- what it is about
- what it is meant to cover (and what topics are meant to be excluded)
- who might find it useful

If the answer to Question 1 is 'No', go directly to Question 3

2. Does it achieve its aims?

Rating this question

No		Partially		Yes
1	2	3	4	5

HINT: Consider whether the publication provides the information it aimed to as outlined in Question 1

3. Is it relevant?

Rating this question

No		Partially		Yes
1	2	3	4	5

HINT: Consider whether:
- the publication addresses the questions that readers might ask
- recommendations and suggestions concerning treatment choices are realistic or appropriate

4. Is it clear what sources of information were used to compile the publication (other than the author or producer)?

Rating this question

No		Partially		Yes
1	2	3	4	5

HINT
- Check whether the main claims or statements made about treatment choices are accompanied by a reference to the sources used as evidence, e.g. a research study or expert opinion
- Look for a means of checking the sources used such as a bibliography/reference list or the addresses of the experts or organizations quoted, or external links to the online sources

Rating note: In order to score a full '5' the publication should fulfil both hints. Lists of **additional** sources of support and information (Question 7) are not necessarily sources of **evidence** for the current publication.

5. Is it clear when the information used or reported in the publication was produced?

Rating this question

No		Partially		Yes
1	2	3	4	5

HINT: Look for:
- dates of the main sources of information used to compile the publication

FIGURE 3.1 **The DISCERN Instrument (cont.)**

- date of any revisions of the publication (but not dates of reprinting in the case of print publications)
- date of publication (copyright date)

Rating note: The hints are placed in order of importance—in order to score a full '5' the dates relating to the first hint should be found.

6. Is it balanced and unbiased?

Rating this question

No		Partially		Yes
1	2	3	4	5

HINT: Look for:
- a clear indication of whether the publication is written from a personal or objective point of view
- evidence that a range of sources of information was used to compile the publication, e.g. more than one research study or expert
- evidence of an external assessment of the publication

Be wary if:
- the publication focuses on the advantages or disadvantages of one particular treatment choice without reference to other possible choices
- the publication relies primarily on evidence from single cases (which may not be typical of people with this condition or of responses to a particular treatment)
- the information is presented in a sensational, emotive or alarmist way

7. Does it provide details of additional sources of support and information?

Rating this question

No		Partially		Yes
1	2	3	4	5

HINT: Look for suggestions for further reading or for details of other organizations providing advice and information about the condition and treatment choices.

8. Does it refer to areas of uncertainty?

Rating this question

No		Partially		Yes
1	2	3	4	5

HINT
- Look for discussion of the gaps in knowledge or differences in expert opinion concerning treatment choices.
- Be wary if the publication implies that a treatment choice affects everyone in the same way, e.g. 100% success rate with a particular treatment

SECTION 2
How good is the quality of information on treatment choices?
N.B. The questions apply to the treatment (or treatments) described **in the publication.**
Self-care is considered a form of treatment throughout this section.

FIGURE 3.1   The DISCERN Instrument (cont.)

9. Does it describe how each treatment works?

Rating this question
No		Partially		Yes
1	2	3	4	5

HINT: Look for a description of how a treatment acts on the body to achieve its effect.

10. Does it describe the benefits of each treatment?

Rating this question
No		Partially		Yes
1	2	3	4	5

HINT: Benefits can include controlling or getting rid of symptoms, preventing recurrence of the condition and eliminating the condition, both short-term and long-term.

11. Does it describe the risks of each treatment?

Rating this question
No		Partially		Yes
1	2	3	4	5

HINT: Risks can include side effects, complications and adverse reactions to treatment, both short-term and long-term.

12. Does it describe what would happen if no treatment is used?

Rating this question
No		Partially		Yes
1	2	3	4	5

HINT: Look for a description of the risks and benefits of postponing treatment, of watchful waiting (i.e. monitoring how the condition progresses without treatment) or of permanently forgoing treatment.

13. Does it describe how the treatment choices affect overall quality of life?

Rating this question
No		Partially		Yes
1	2	3	4	5

HINT: Look for:
- description of the effects of the treatment choices on day-to-day activity
- description of the effects of the treatment choices on relationships with family, friends and carers

14. Is it clear that there may be more than one possible treatment choice?

Rating this question
No		Partially		Yes
1	2	3	4	5

HINT: Look for:
- a description of who is most likely to benefit from each treatment choice mentioned, and under what circumstances
- suggestions of alternatives to consider or investigate further (including choices not fully described in the publication) before deciding whether to select or reject a particular treatment choice

FIGURE | 3.1

The DISCERN Instrument (cont.)

Rating this question

	No		Partially		Yes

15. Does it provide support for shared decision-making?   1   2   3   4   5

HINT Look for suggestions of things to discuss with family, friends, doctors or other health professionals concerning treatment choices.

SECTION 3. Overall Rating of the Publication

Rating this question

	No		Partially		Yes

16. Based on the answers to all of the above questions, rate the overall quality of the publication as a source of information about treatment choices   1   2   3   4   5

Rating this question

Low		**Moderate**		**High**
Serious or extensive shortcomings		Potentially important but not serious shortcomings		Minimal shortcomings
1	2	3	4	5

Copyright British Library and the University of Oxford 1997
Used with permission of Sasha Shepperd, MSc, D.Phil

Levels of evidence

When examining the written word, consider whether the materials are based on research or opinion. When ideas are presented in published materials, readers often assume them to be factual, but errors can and do occur in publications. Also, published materials can range in quality from editorials and letters to formal research studies involving human subjects. The rigor of any scientific effort significantly affects the reliability and validity of the results of the study and the ability to generalize the results to other populations and settings. Therefore, it is very important to assess the type of article you are reviewing. Determine and critique the research methods using a structured evaluation process (see Chapter 5 for more details on critiquing research articles).

Assessing the level or strength of the evidence has become a much more formalized process since the inception of evidence-based medicine. Several rating systems have emerged and, at present, groups involved in evidence-based efforts report levels of evidence and/or grades of recommendation. Initially, the work in evidence-based medicine and the availability of extensive research publications resulted in levels of evidence that primarily related to research articles. In contrast, when rating scales were first developed for nursing, there were many fewer published research studies available to review and evaluate. This resulted in rating scales for certain topics that started with the lowest level, which included opinion-based articles, and higher levels, which included randomized control studies. Various rating scales continue to be used today in nursing as the research base continues to develop and expand.

Levels of evidence become very important when reviewing or developing clinical practice guidelines. Such classification systems help clinicians and others rate the quality and rigor of the literature. Clinicians first must determine what rating scale has been used or will be used for a particular effort. Several of these classifications exist and may include from three to eight or more levels (West et al., 2002). In the United States, the Agency for Healthcare Research and Quality (AHRQ) serves as the recognized authority regarding the assessment of clinical research, and the table below highlights their rating scale.

FIGURE 3.2 Levels of evidence

AHRQ levels of evidence	Classification
Meta-analysis of multiple well-designed controlled studies	1A
Well-designed randomized controlled trials	1
Well-designed non-randomized controlled trial (quasi-experiments)	2
Observational studies with controls (retrospective studies, interrupted time studies, case-control studies, cohort studies, with controls)	3
Observational studies without controls (cohort studies without controls and case series)	4

Grades of recommendation reflect the level or strength of the evidence and provide guidance about whether to include a particular action. These types of classification systems can guide the decisions of guideline developers. For example, the evidence may be

- good or fair
- for or against a certain intervention
- conflicting
- insufficient

Different guideline developers may provide these grades of recommendation within a particular guideline to help guide clinical practice. In this way, a clinician is clear about why a particular recommendation for practice is made.

An ongoing international collaboration focuses on improving the quality and effectiveness of clinical practice guidelines. This group has established a framework for determining the quality of guidelines for diagnoses, health promotion, treatments, or clinical interventions. This effort is called AGREE, which stands for "Appraisal of Guidelines Research and Evaluation" (*www.agreecollaboration.org*). The AGREE instrument is intended to be used with new, existing, or updated guidelines and is generally used by groups as part of a formal assessment of a specific guideline.

Learning how to evaluate clinical practice guidelines and learning to rate the evidence are integral components of implementing evidence-based practice. Clinicians, however, need education and practice to use these tools. Accessing various resources that provide evidence-based practice guidelines or education about using evidence can provide nursing education and help improve patient care. Nurses working in evidence-based practice councils can team up, explore these materials together, and practice new skills. Learning about and working with the evidence can be fun and helpful to nurses' ongoing efforts to provide high-quality, evidence-based care.

Practice exercises

1. Visit the National Guideline Clearinghouse (*www.ngc.gov*) and find an evidence-based protocol that relates to a topic or issue of interest.

2. Conduct a search on PubMed and narrow or broaden the topic based on the number of articles identified. Use the menus to limit the search to articles since 2000.

3. Perform a Web search on the same topic, and identify the number and types of responses you obtain.

4. Visit one of the Web sites that focuses on evidence-based practice in nursing. Explore the various resources and evidence-based practice guidelines on that site.

5. Review nursing policies and procedures at your organization and see whether the reference lists include research articles.

References

Nicoll, L.H., & Beyea, S.C. (2000). Working with staff around evidence-based practice: The next generation of research utilization. *Seminars in Perioperative Nursing, 9,* 133–142.

West, S., King, V., Carey, T. S., et. al. (2002). Systems to rate the strength of scientific evidence. *Evidence Report/Technology Assessment No. 47.* AHRQ Publication No. 02-E016.

Further reading

Craig, J.V., & Smyth, R.L. (Eds.). (2002). *The Evidence-Based Practice Manual for Nurses*. New York: Churchill Livingstone.

Malloch, K. & Porter-O'Grady, T. (Eds.). (2005). *Introduction to Evidence-Based Practice in Nursing and Health Care*. Boston: Jones & Bartlett Publishers.

Strauss, S.E., Richardson, W.S., Glasziou, P.R. & Haynes, B. (2005). *Evidence-Based Medicine*. 3rd ed. New York: Churchill Livingstone.

Evidence-based practice becomes a reality

By Julie Shocksnider, RNC, MS, CCE

Learning objectives

After reading this chapter, the participant should be able to
- identify a model of evidence-based practice (EBP)
- discuss approaches to integrate evidence into nursing practice

Questions for nurses

When implementing evidence-based practice, nurses may consider questions such as the following:

- Do I believe that using the best practices in care will result in the highest quality outcomes for patients and families?

- How do I know what I know about nursing practice? Where and when did I learn about various nursing interventions? How current is my nursing knowledge?

- Are my nursing decisions based upon myths, traditions, experience, authority, trial and error, ritual, or scientific knowledge? (Carper, 1988)

Questions for nursing leadership
Nursing leadership must strongly support both making changes and adopting evidence-based practice. Questions to ask of nursing leaders include the following:

- Does my chief nurse executive believe in and demonstrate commitment to evidence-based practice?

- How does the chief nurse executive demonstrate support?

- How does the organizational culture support evidence-based practice?

- What budget exists to support evidence-based nursing practice?

- What resources are offered within the nursing library and electronically?

- How is information about evidence-based nursing practice currently being disseminated to the bedside nurse?

- Are we an ANCC Magnet Recognition Program® (MRP) facility or are we applying for designation, and does adequate support for nursing research exist?

Match your organization's culture

Each healthcare organization has a unique culture and approach to evidence-based practice, and EBP implementation should match this culture. Despite this variation, when first starting out, all nurses must have the opportunity to learn about and participate in related initiatives. Additionally, all nurses must be made aware that this effort is valued and important.

Also note that the resources available to implement EBP may vary due to the organization's size and financial status.

Assess the organization

When conducting an organizational assessment, survey nurses' knowledge, attitudes, beliefs, and views regarding nursing research and evidence-based practice. Doing so allows you to establish the foundation for discussions and efforts related to evidence-based nursing practice. Surveying staff members also provides opportunities to identify potential champions in each clinical area. Ask the following questions during this survey:

- How does this organization promote evidence-based nursing practice?

- Is the library adequate to promote research in nursing practice?

- In this organization, does nursing consistently use research to guide practice?

- Is evidence-based practice in nursing viewed as important?

- Is evidence easy to obtain in the healthcare organization? What other data sources exist?

- Do nurses currently use evidence in their practice?

- Are nurses interested in conducting nursing research?

- Would nurses like more education about evidence-based practice?

- What are nurses' beliefs regarding evidence-based practice?

- Do nurses believe that policies, guidelines, and procedures serve as key strategies to incorporate evidence into their practice?

- Do nurses know how to obtain evidence and perform literature searches?

- Can nurses interpret the literature and research if they can access it?

- Do nurses believe that an evidence-based practice model can be used within their healthcare organization?

- Are nurses interested in serving on a nursing research or evidence-based practice council?

Open-ended statements such as the following might help in this process as well:

- As a nurse, I would use evidence-based strategies in my practice if . . .
- It would help my practice if . . .
- I would be willing to serve on a nursing research or evidence-based practice council if . . .

Should an organization choose to use a survey, the results may be analyzed and summarized by the new nursing research or evidence-based practice (EBP) council. Note that it is not necessary for an organization to develop or modify its own survey to assess the knowledge, attitudes, and beliefs of nurses about research and evidence-based practice. In fact, the first role of the nursing research or EBP council can be conducting a literature search to identify potential surveys. This project can serve as a first step in the research process and help involve group members in using the evidence to make decisions.

Create a nursing research council or evidence-based practice council

To review and analyze the data collected by the survey, form a nursing evidence-based practice council or a nursing research council.

Identify council members

Identify council members from the survey process. They may include bedside nurses, managers, educators, clinical nurse specialists, and other master's-prepared nurses.

Specifically, include a nurse researcher, and consider asking a research physician or another practitioner experienced in research to serve as a member or otherwise support the council's initiatives. A librarian may be a helpful council member, so encourage one to join. Also note that a physical therapist, dietary, respiratory therapist, or pharmacist with research experience or interest might join on a per diem or regular basis, depending on the work of the group and the structure of the organization.

Organize the first meeting

Once you create your council, determine a date, time, and comfortable location for its first meeting, and send out invitations that include an agenda and that encourage participants to come with ideas for the nursing research council. If the budget supports it, hold a luncheon to welcome potential members and encourage attendance. The convener of the council should work with unit leadership to make sure that staff nurses have release time to attend the meetings.

Create an agenda

The agenda for the research or evidence-based practice council's first meeting could include some of the following topics:

- Welcome and introduce participants (chief nurse executive)

- Discuss results of the nursing research survey (if already conduced)
    - What do nurses desire and need to support evidence-based research?
    - How can evidence-based practice be supported and advanced based upon the findings from the survey?
    - What would be the most helpful education plan?
    - Identify key clinical issues or problems for evidence-based activities.

- Vote on co-chairs of the council and define their responsibilities

- Discuss current evidence-based initiatives

- Discuss models for evidence-based practice, and determine which one is the best fit for the organization

- Discuss the council's purpose

- Discuss the council's role in reviewing and critiquing nursing research proposals

- Develop a nursing research policy

- Open discussion of other topics

- Set date/time of meetings for the year (initially schedule monthly)

Create a list of members, including names, titles, and contact information, and determine how information about the meetings will be disseminated. Also, take minutes and consider creating a notebook or file for nursing evidence-based practice initiatives. Make clear assignments with due dates to ensure results. Council members also may consider developing bylaws for the council and establishing other polices and procedures. Typically, nursing research councils develop both procedures for reviewing nursing research proposals and guidelines for the approval process.

Nursing research or evidence-based practice policy

One goal of the research or evidence-based practice council could be to develop a policy or guideline related to proposed nursing research efforts. Ideally, the policy would include a purpose that addresses the importance of nursing research and evidence-based practice.

The policy should contain clear guidelines on conducting research—specifically, it should outline procedures to protect the rights of human subjects. The research council also needs to clarify its relationship to the organization's institutional review board (IRB).

If its intent is to guide nurse researchers, the policy should address which procedures need to be followed to get unit or departmental approval before starting a research project. It should address the role of nurse researchers who are not affiliated with the organization. It also should address procedures for the review of any nursing research proposal. (See Figure 4.1: Sample nursing research policy.)

Purpose and role of the council

Council members must consider carefully the group's core values and functions. Identify them in the early phases of the council's formation and review and revise them periodically. Beyond reviewing nursing research proposals, the council may limit its role to be that of education and consultation. Other functions to consider include

- reviewing and critiquing research and evidence-based practice guidelines
- collaborating with nurses who conduct quality improvement initiatives to promote the use of evidence
- sponsoring a research symposium or roundtable discussions for nurses
- developing nursing research projects
- answering staff nurses' research questions
- encouraging and supporting evidence-based practice

The council's role should be consistent with the organizational and departmental priorities and resources. Having the council actually conduct research might be a better fit to an organization that has access to a qualified nurse researcher in some capacity, whereas another organization may need to focus on helping staff nurses ask questions about their own practices. Clarifying the functions of the group will help focus the work plan.

FIGURE 4.1   **Sample nursing research policy**

Dartmouth-Hitchcock Medical Center
Lebanon, New Hampshire
Office of Professional Nursing

GUIDELINES FOR REVIEW OF
RESEARCH PROPOSALS INVOLVING NURSES

Research involving nurses in roles as investigators, subjects, care givers, or data collectors must be reviewed by the Committee for the Protection of Human Subjects (CPHS), the institutional review board for DHMC. Prior to submission to the CPHS, all research proposals must undergo scientific review by a departmental research group or other designated authority.

The Office of Professional Nursing conducts the departmental scientific review for nurse investigators or for studies where the subjects are DHMC nurses. Nurse investigators may elect to go through the research committees of departments of Dartmouth Medical School if they desire. It is the objective of the Nursing Research Office to assist nurse investigators with the research proposal development and approval process.

Nurse Researchers must either be employees of DHMC or Dartmouth College or collaborate with a researcher who meets the employment criteria of CPHS.

To initiate the steps of the review process in the Office of Professional Nursing, the investigator contacts the Nursing Research Coordinator.

I. Departmental Scientific Review (Nursing)

    A. Investigators are encouraged to contact the Director of Nursing Research or the Nursing Research Coordinator in the early stages of proposal development. A copy of the guidelines for the scientific and administrative review process will be provided and time frames for accomplishing the review within investigator deadlines will be discussed.

    B. Investigator presents four copies of the research proposal, an abstract of the proposal following the format required by the CPHS and a copy of the CPHS cover sheet to the Nursing Research Coordinator. The proposal should include

        1. Background information sufficient to establish the significance of studying this problem.
        2. Description of the problem and objectives of the study.
        3. Description of research plan: sample selection, instruments, procedures.
        4. Projected plan for analysis and interpretation of data.
        5. Consent forms where appropriate.
        6. Data collection instruments, questionnaires, and cover letters where appropriate. (Should be attached to proposal.)
        7. Estimate of numbers of patients/staff to be involved.
        8. Estimate of time per subject and total staff nurse time involved.
        9. A letter of support from the Director(s) (or designee) of the department(s) involved.
        10. Time frame for conduct of study.

FIGURE 4.1   Sample nursing research policy (cont.)

11. Potential implications of study for nursing practice.

12. Plan for communicating final report.

C. If a proposal is being submitted by a student, a letter from the faculty member who is the primary advisor on the project must accompany the proposal submission. The letter must identify how the faculty member can be reached by letter and by telephone and must contain the faculty member's endorsement of the project.

D. The proposal will be reviewed within 10 days of submission by three nurses selected by the Nursing Research Coordinator.

Reviewers will be master's-prepared nurses selected from the following groups in order of priority:

1. Clinical Nurse Specialist, if study falls within area of expertise.

2. Nursing Director if study would be conducted on units for which they are administratively responsible.

3. Other master's (or doctorally) prepared nurses within DHMC whose area of research or clinical expertise would qualify them to review the proposal.

E. Reviewers will complete the Scientific Review of Research Proposal forms, or, if appropriate, the Administrative Review of Research Proposals, and return them to the Nursing Research Coordinator. Approval of research proposals will be dependent on the following criteria:

1. The problem is relevant and timely.

2. The research design is appropriate and logical.

3. The rights and safety of patients and staff have been adequately safeguarded.

4. There is potential benefit to patients, staff, or the nursing profession.

5. The study will not interfere with or compromise existing programs of care.

6. The study is feasible in terms of staff time, space, and/or materials required.

7. There is a plan to share the study results with the nursing staff and appropriate others.

F. The outcomes of the review for scientific merit will result in one of the following actions:

1. Full approval

2. Approval pending review of revisions.

3. Recommendation of revisions of study plan to enhance protection of human subjects, scientific merit, and feasibility.

The Nursing Research Coordinator will assist the investigator in addressing any revision requested by the review panel. Once any outstanding questions have been addressed, the Director of Nursing Research will sign the CPHS coversheet. The proposal will be returned to the investigator after the signature of approval from the Director of Nursing Research has been obtained. Allow 10 to 14 days for the review process.

II. Human Subjects Review

A. The Committee for the Protection of Human Subjects (CPHS) is the institutional review board at DHMC. Investigators

FIGURE 4.1 **Sample nursing research policy (cont.)**

should contact the IRB Administrator to obtain the most recent versions of the CPHS cover sheet and informed consent forms. Forms are also available on the CPHS Web page.

B. After the research proposal has been approved by the Office of Professional Nursing, it is the responsibility of the investigator to submit the research proposal to the Committee for the Protection of Human Subjects (DHMC use: CPHS mailbox in mailroom).

C. Data collection may begin when the investigator submits the letter of approval from the CPHS to the Nursing Research Coordinator's office, and the letter of approval with a copy of the proposal to the directors of any units on which the study will take place.

D. It is the responsibility of the investigator to keep the Office of Professional Nursing apprised of the status of the study including submissions of copies of the CPHS Annual Renewal and Termination forms.

III. When the investigator is also a student

A. When doing a research project as part of an academic requirement, the student is responsible for meeting the often different criteria set by both his or her school and DHMC. It is advisable to contact the Nursing Research Coordinator early in the process of proposal development for guidance in understanding the standards used for evaluating research proposals at DHMC.

B. The student should be aware of the time requirements of the review process and allow for possible revisions.

Source: Dartmouth-Hitchcock Medical Center. Used with permission.

The council may decide that its initial work effort will focus on making polices and procedures evidence-based. This can be a great place to start, as it helps embed evidence in the care nurses provide each day. In addition, policies and procedures are clinically relevant and can transform research findings into practice. If an organization is considering pursuing MRP designation, this focus will help in those efforts by ensuring that policies and standards of care incorporate research findings and evidence-based guidelines. Once policies and procedures have been revised, the council also could conduct clinical evaluations and assess the effectiveness of practice changes. In this way, quality indicators and outcomes can be linked to evidence-based practice.

Tips for Success

The EBP or nursing research council will enjoy
most success if it has a clear purpose and function.

Models of evidence-based nursing practice

No one model of evidence-based practice is a perfect fit for all nursing departments and all evidence-based nursing efforts. A healthcare organization may already have established multidisciplinary evidence-based practice groups, and nursing may decide to use a similar model and approach. Another organization may decide to develop its own model or adapt an existing model. At an initial meeting, council members could review and evaluate existing models and determine which would be the best fit. This strategy helps council members learn more about approaches to evidence-based practice while choosing a model that will help guide their efforts.

Numerous models have been developed and used by experts in evidence-based practice in different clinical settings. Individuals or organizations interested in learning about these models should conduct a literature search. Below are a few of the models that have been described in the literature:

- The Academic Center for Evidence-Based Nursing (ACE) Star Model of Knowledge Transformation® (*www.acestar.uthscsa.edu/Learn_model.htm*).

- The University of Colorado's evidence-based multidisciplinary clinical practice model (Goode & Piedalue, 1999).

- Rosswurm and Larrabee's model for change to evidence-based practice (Rosswurm & Larrabee, 1999).

- The Iowa Model of Evidence-Based Practice (*www.uihealthcare.com/depts/nursing/rqom/ evidencebasedpractice/iowamodel.html*).

Each of these approaches or components from more than one model may help an organization's evidence-based efforts. Members of research or evidence-based practice councils should evaluate these and any other identified models for their fit to the setting. If no model is a perfect fit, the group could decide to adapt a model or create a new one.

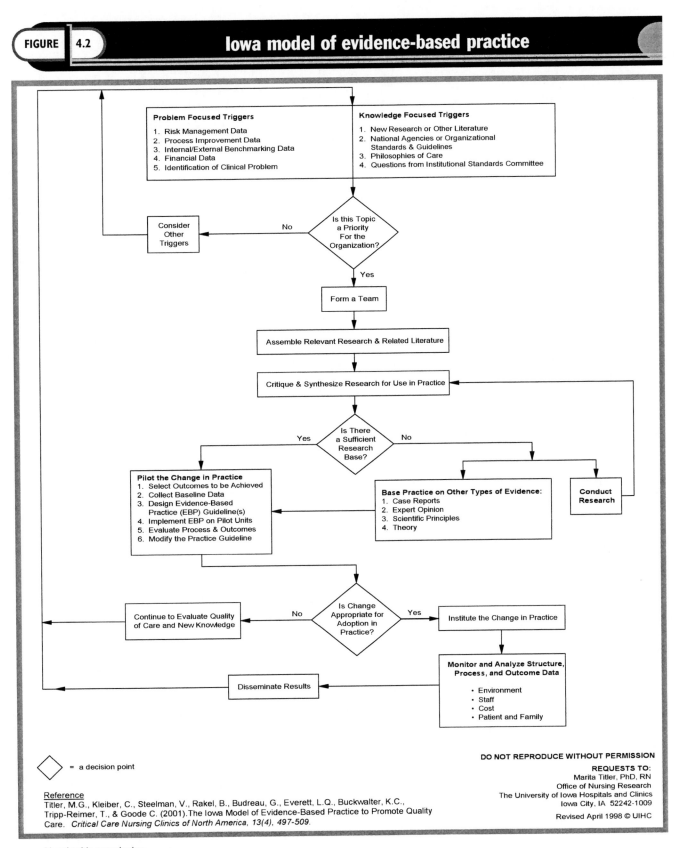

FIGURE 4.2 — **Iowa model of evidence-based practice**

Used with permission

Iowa Model of Evidence-Based Practice

Consider as a framework the Iowa Model of Evidence-Based Practice. Within the model, evidence-based practice starts with identifying either knowledge- or problem-focused triggers. It provides a flow diagram to support a sequential approach and key decision points. It also guides the processes that integrate evidence into practice and helps make decisions when research findings are not available to guide practice.

This clearly presented model provides a simple and straightforward framework that most clinicians will find easy to follow and a fit to their practice environment (Titler, et al., 2001). (See Figure 4.2: Iowa Model of Evidence-Based Practice.)

Research champions

When implementing EBP, identify individuals who can champion and promote evidence-based practice. These individuals can serve on the research or evidence-based practice council and can champion evidence-based practice within their clinical departments. Having a champion on every nursing unit can help to develop capacity for evidence-based practice throughout the entire nursing organization.

The best champions might not be immediately obvious, so look everywhere. For example, a physical therapist might edit his or her professional magazine, or a librarian may have completed a research project. The staff members who work in the Quality Department might be interested in conducting research or developing collaborative projects between quality improvement efforts and nursing research initiatives (Mateo & Kirchhoff, 1999). Other champions can include nurses who are enrolled in research courses as they pursue advanced studies. Their participation and involvement might be extremely helpful and bring energy and enthusiasm to the group.

Tips for Success

Unit-based EBP champions can help build support and
understanding among all nurses.

Education on evidence-based practice

There are many ways to educate an organization about evidence-based practice. Often, nurses first must learn the basics of evidence-based practice, so an introduction to the topic can be crucial. Try collaborating with the nursing education department—educators may be able to identify the best educational strategies to achieve the desired results.

Strategies to present and explain EBP include self-study packets either in hard copies or online. One organization developed Web-delivered research-based staff education and found this method to be effective and flexible (Belcher & Vonderhaar, 2005). Another organization used the train-the-trainer strategy in its efforts to build capacity for evidence-based practice (Newhouse, Dearbolt, Poe, Pugh, & White, 2005). Nursing grand rounds offer another avenue for disseminating information about evidence-based practices.

Presentation topics could include evidence-based information or focus specifically on answering the question, "What is evidence-based nursing?" Clinical topics might provide an avenue for research dissemination and be interesting to nurses. Nurses will appreciate being offered continuing education contact hours for these educational programs, and it may increase their attendance at the various sessions. Also note that varying your approach may encourage more nurses to participate. All nurses should learn how to use the PICO format to ask clinical questions. The acronym means

P = Patient population
I = Intervention or topic of interest
C = Comparison that will be conducted
O = Outcome

This questioning framework helps nurses ask pertinent clinical questions and helps them focus on asking the right question.

To learn more about using PICO to ask good research questions, visit the resources at

- *www.urmc.rochester.edu/hslt/miner/resources/evidence_based/index.cfm*
- *http://ebling.library.wisc.edu/classes_tutorials/coursepages/pharm675/PICO.pdf*
- *www.studentbmj.com/back_issues/0902/education/313.html*

Note that orientation for recent nurse graduates or experienced nurses is the perfect time for the chair of the research council to discuss nursing research and evidence-based practice with all newly employed staff. Educators and clinical nurse specialists can promote evidence-based practice during annual competencies on each unit. Create a link between research findings, education, and competency development to make evidence-based practice a reality.

Tips for Success

During orientation is the perfect time to get new employees used to the organization's focus on evidence-based practice.

Dissemination of evidence-based practice efforts

Make the efforts of the research council known throughout the organization. There are many ways to do so, and again, the organization's culture may support one strategy more than others. Some healthcare organizations have established a research or evidence-based practice bulletin board, which can be as simple as a cork board on each of the nursing units with a nursing research title or a specially created board with holders for handouts.

A nursing research "corner" on each clinical unit can serve as another method of distributing and communicating research topics to the nurses. This corner might be a shelf or table within each unit's break room where articles, newsletters, and other materials can be distributed. The council minutes can be distributed via e-mail, via hardcopy, or on a research board/corner. Access to a nursing research "hotline" provides an easy way for nurses to communicate with the council regarding evidence-based questions or concerns.

Try using a research newsletter to distribute highlights from meeting minutes and to disseminate other evidence-based practice updates. It could include some of the following headings:

- Evidence-based practice online resources and how to access these resources
- Examples of evidence-based practice
- Research term of the month
- Research and the MRP initiative
- Update from the evidence-based nursing council and meeting dates/times

- Overview of research initiatives within your organizations
- Facilitators and barriers of evidence-based practice

The newsletter can be in a print or an electronic format and can be distributed or posted on the bulletin board. Finding a strategy that is consistent with organizational culture and that will grab staff nurses' attention will prove most helpful.

Developing and setting up a nursing research poster board can help council members periodically connect with staff members. Placing a poster where staff nurses eat lunch or in another high-traffic area increases the chances that it will be read. Research games, such as a crossword puzzle or bingo, also can be used to encourage participation with small prizes, candy, or handouts as incentives. Be creative, and try to connect with as many potentially interested staff nurses as possible to build enthusiasm for evidence-based practice.

Supporting inquiry

Provide nurses with opportunities to come together through journal clubs (discussed in detail in Chapter 5), grand rounds, informal unit gatherings, and staff meetings. In these forums, nurses can discuss research topics such as how to critique a nursing research article. The research or evidence-based practice council might create or adapt an existing evaluation form to use when critiquing the literature. Such a form will help nurses evaluate articles using a structured framework.

Using multiple approaches helps create an evidence-based nursing practice environment. Not all nurses will be prepared at the doctoral level or will want to focus on research, but all nurses should know how to be consumers of nursing research. They want the best possible care for their patients as well as for themselves, and becoming a savvy consumer of nursing research helps them use research findings to improve patient outcomes.

With the support of the nursing leadership team and other more experienced nurse consumers or researchers, nurses can obtain, evaluate, interpret, and implement research findings into clinical practice. Building capacity for evidence-based practice is the first step in the process. When staff nurses become engaged in the process and see evidence of its benefits, both patients and nursing staff see positive outcomes. Enjoy the evidence-based practice pathway—improving patient care and practice environments is fun for all involved.

Practice exercises

1. Determine whether your organization or nursing department has a group that focuses on evidence-based practice. Learn more about the group and the focus of their efforts. Are they implementing evidence-based guidelines or conducting research?

2. Learn more about each of the evidence-based practice models, and decide which one makes the most sense to you. Consider which one you think would be most useful to your colleagues. Consider why you chose that one.

3. When you attend continuing education sessions, ask for a reference list and try to determine whether research findings were included in the speaker's presentation.

4. If your organization has a nursing research council, ask to attend as a guest and learn more about the work efforts of the group. Review their bylaws and minutes.

5. Determine local resources for learning more about nursing research. Are continuing education offerings available? Is there a local college that offers nursing research courses?

References

Belcher, J. V. R. & Vonderhaar, K.J. (2005) Web-delivered research-based nursing staff education for seeking Magnet status. Journal of Nursing Administration, 35 (9), 382–386.

Carper, B.A. (1988). Response to perspectives on knowing: a model of nursing knowledge. *Scholarly Inquiry for Nursing Practice,* 2 (2), 141–144.

Goode, C. J., & Piedalae, F. (1999). Evidence-based clinical practice. *Journal of Nursing Administration,* 29 (6), 15–21.

Mateo, M.A. & Kirchhoff, K.T. (1999). *Using and conducting nursing research in the clinical setting.* Philadelphia: W.B. Saunders Company.

Newhouse, R., Dearbolt, S., Poe, S., Pugh, L.C., & White, K.M. (2005). Evidence-based practice. *Journal of Nursing Administration, 35* (3), 35–40.

Rosswurm, M. A. & Larrabee, J.H.. (1999). A model to change to evidence-based practice. *Image: Journal of Nursing Scholarship.*

Titler, M.G., Kleiber, C., Steelman, V.J., Rakel, B.A., Budreau, G., Everett, L.Q., et al. (2001). The Iowa model of evidence-based practice to promote quality care. *Critical Care Nursing Clinical of North America, 13* (4), 497–509.

Davies, B.L. (2002). Sources and models for moving research evidence into clinical practice. *Journal of Obstetric, Gynecologic and Neonatal Nursing, 31* (5), 558–562.

Stetler, C.B. (2001). Updating the Stetler model of research utilization to facilitate evidence-based practice. *Nursing Outlook, 49* (6), 272–279.

Online evidence-based practice resources:
www.evidencebasednursing.com
www.ahcpr.gov/clinic/epcix.htm
www.nursingsociety.org

Journal clubs

Learning objectives

After reading this chapter, the participant should be able to
- identify why journal clubs are an effective way to start EBP
- discuss guidelines for successful journal clubs

What are journal clubs?

A journal club consists of a group of nurses (or other members of the healthcare team) who meet regularly to discuss and critique research articles appearing in scientific journals. As discussed briefly in Chapter 2, creating one is a good way to get started in evidence-based nursing practice. Journal clubs provide nurses with the opportunity and skills to read and critically evaluate current research and to determine its applicability to their practice area.

The journal club's goals may vary by setting. In the beginning, a goal might be to learn how to appraise research and other evidence-based practice articles critically. Later goals may include keeping up to date with the current research in the field or evaluating current practice based on the evidence related to a particular issue.

Tips for Success

Set manageable goals for journal clubs. Start with a basic question, and then progress to more complicated projects once proficiency increases.

Often a master's-prepared clinical nurse specialist, nurse practitioner, or educator facilitates the journal club. Depending on the setting, however, any nurse or other healthcare provider with the knowledge and interest could act in that role. All educational levels of nursing preparation should be encouraged to participate, and nurses who participate in journal clubs often become champions for evidence-based practice in their settings. One hospital reported using the journal club as a way to help staff nurses develop their critical thinking skills (Speers, 1999).

According to Phillips and Glasziou (2004), the most successful journal clubs have a designated facilitator who helps lead the discussion and keeps the group focused. Other roles, which can be rotated among participants, include a presenter, a scribe to take notes, and someone to provide administrative support.

Tips for Success

Identify a facilitator who can keep the group focused and meetings on track.

There are many approaches to journal clubs, so it is important to identify which formats will work best in your organization. Some authors recommend an optimal number of participants for journal club members. For instance, Klapper (2001) recommends having six to 20 regular members, whereas Dyckoff (2004) reports success with inviting all staff nurses in the institution and having about 40 attend each monthly meeting. Use the general guidelines below as a framework to get started.

Guidelines for journal clubs

1. Determine nurses' level of interest. Notices placed on bulletin boards or electronic lists can provide the goals of the journal club and help recruit members.
2. Establish the support and participation of nursing leadership early on in the development phase to make organizational issues easier to address.
3. Meeting schedules should be set up ahead of time and align with staff availability. Lunchtime or change-of-shift are two logical options, but also consider the night shift. Determine meeting frequency by each particular setting.
4. Choose a convenient meeting location.
5. Identify journal articles for discussion. As discussed in Chapter 3, availability of electronic databases makes literature searches easy to perform if the resources are available for access within your organization.

6. Select topics that are clinically relevant to the members of the group. Journal clubs work best if the nurses identify research topics that are relevant to their practice setting. In the early phase of the journey to EBP, nurses must become confident, proficient, and competent in finding articles and in conducting a formal critique of nursing research articles. As their knowledge level progresses, identifying specific topics and asking relevant clinical questions for evidence-based practice will evolve.

7. Distribute copies of the selected article and any critique guidelines in advance to allow enough time for nurses to read them before the scheduled meeting. In organizations with electronic library resources, the article link may be e-mailed to participants.

8. The journal club can be interdisciplinary as long as it focuses on nursing practice. According to Klapper (2001), including members from diverse clinical backgrounds promotes the exchange of different perspectives, but it may make focusing difficult.

9. Have fun, and encourage all to participate.

10. At the end of each session, evaluate the journal club and select a topic for the next meeting.

Alternative approaches to traditional journal clubs

Some barriers to creating a traditional journal club include lack of time to attend one-hour sessions and the difficulty of involving nurses from all shifts. One innovative solution was reported by Pasek and Zack (2004). On their very busy pediatric intensive care unit, the APN facilitator made herself available to nurses in a very central location and covered a few aspects of the article discussion at a time. She repeated this several times in each shift to accommodate nurses' availability as they provided patient care. With some creativity and flexibility, journal clubs can work in even the busiest settings.

Public forums

Many scientific journals now offer their own versions of a journal club in which a journal article—whether published in that journal or not—is critiqued. *The American Journal of Critical Care* features an AJCC Journal Club article and a Web link to questions and article discussion points that can be found online (*www.ajcconline.org*). The Oncology Nursing Forum selects a clinically relevant article and provides specific ideas to facilitate journal club discussion (*www.ons.org/publications*). Individual nurses can use these questions as well.

Other journals, such as the *Archives of Pediatric and Adolescent Medicine*, conduct critical analyses of a study reported in each issue in the "Evidence-Based Journal Club." The ACP Journal Club (*www.acpjc.org*), published bimonthly by the American College of Physicians, selects original studies and systematic reviews related to internal medicine from more than 100 journals and summarizes them for practice. Many of these studies may be relevant to nursing practice as well.

Learning how to critique the nursing literature

Once nurses decide they want to form a journal club, they often wonder how to determine an appropriate research article and how to begin critiquing one.

The first step is to select articles that are research-based and from a peer-reviewed journal. Other suggested guidelines for selecting appropriate literature include the following:

- Articles should be no more than five years old
- Studies from medical journals should be limited and used only if the topic relates to a nursing issue
- Either quantitative or qualitative research articles are appropriate for review
- Use of secondary sources or nursing textbooks must be avoided
- When possible, select articles with a comparable patient population
- Be sure the article focuses on nursing interventions, not medical interventions

The above guidelines are only intended to serve as a general framework. Note that the article selected must be appropriate for nurses who are in the novice to advanced beginner stage of EBP knowledge development.

Nurses can learn the EBP process and how to critique research studies in stages. Initially, select research studies that do not bog down the group in complex statistical tests. If the article does have complex statistics, seek additional guidance with that aspect of the review if it is beyond the scope of the facilitator. The critique and discussion will be much more meaningful if the article selected is relevant to the group and addresses a current clinical problem.

Guidelines for the critique of nursing research articles

The overall goal of a research critique is to evaluate a study's merits and its applicability to clinical practice. A research critique goes beyond a review or summary of a study, and it carefully appraises a study's strengths and limitations. By evaluating a study's component parts, the critique should assess objectively a study's validity and significance.

As discussed in the previous chapters, several guidelines for the appraisal of evidence—in the form of meta-analyses, systematic reviews, and clinical practice guidelines—have been published in print and online. In addition to nursing research textbooks, several published guidelines for how to review single research studies can help nurses in their journal club endeavors (Brown, 1999). See Chapter 3 for online resources for evidence-based practice. The following resources specifically target the critical appraisal of research studies:

- Critical appraisal tools developed by the Critical Appraisal Skills Program, (suitable for all types of studies) NHS Trust-Public Health Resource Unit. (*www.phru.nhs.uk/casp/critical_appraisal_tools.htm)*

- Critical appraisal worksheets in the EBM Toolbox, Center for Evidence-Based Medicine at Oxford (*www.cebm.net*).

- Users' Guide to Evidence-Based Practice. Site maintained by the Canadian Centre for Health Evidence (*www.cche.net/usersguides/start.asp*). (Originally published in the *Journal of the American Medical Asociation.*)

Tips for Success

Choose articles that are research-based and from a peer-reviewed journal.

The level of discussion at the initial journal club meetings will depend on the facilitator's knowledge base. Nurses who have completed graduate-level research courses will be able to guide the group so that all questions can be answered and discussed. It may not be possible, however, to have a registered nurse with a master's degree serve as a facilitator for every journal club. If this is the case in your organization, consider limiting how many journal clubs meet to ensure adequate mentorship. Another choice is to have baccalaureate-prepared nurses serve as facilitators and understand that, in the beginning, certain questions may pose a challenge to the group. In that case, the group should agree to discuss as many of the questions as possible and to skip over questions they find difficult. The facilitator can then follow up with someone who can clarify the difficult areas of the critique. With experience, educational sessions, and mentoring, nurses' knowledge and confidence levels will continue to increase. Evidence-based practice, like any new skill, takes practice. Journal clubs are a great way to learn the skills necessary to evaluate the evidence and to decide whether it's applicable to specific practice areas.

Beyea and Nicoll (1997) published a simple guide of 10 questions to use when reading and discussing a research article. The questions can be used to assess the quality of the study and to determine its applicability to clinical practice. This tool is an effective introduction to critiquing and is especially helpful to the novice consumer of research. (See Figure 5.1)

FIGURE 5.1	Ten questions for a research report review

10 questions for critiquing	Clarifying points
1. What is the research question?	Is it understandable? Can you paraphrase it?
2. What is the basis for this research question?	To what aspect of nursing practice, education, or theory does it relate?
3. Why is this research question important?	Is it clinically relevant?
4. How was the research question studied?	What methods were used?
5. Does the study make sense?	Does the method used match the research question?
6. Were the correct subjects selected for the study?	How were they selected? Did they obtain informed consent?
7. Was the research question answered?	Describe the findings.
8. Does the answer make sense?	Do the findings support the hypothesis?
9. What is next?	Research leaves many unanswered questions. What would be the next question to explore?
10. So what?	Is this study and its findings relevant to clinical practice?

Practice exercises

1. Meet with a group of registered nurses from your nursing unit or practice setting. Generate a list of topics that they would like to investigate as part of EBP.

2. Based on the generated topics, select a few articles from the nursing literature for discussion and critique them at a future journal club. How long did it take you to find some articles?

3. Identify potential journal club facilitators. Have them review the guidelines for article critique presented in this chapter. Are they comfortable in assisting registered nurses in the critique process? If not, who will provide them with an educational review?

References

Beyea, S.C., & Nicoll, L.H. (1997). Ten questions that will get you through any research report. *AORN Journal, 65* (5), 978–979.

Brown, S. J. (1999). Appraising findings from single original studies. In *Knowledge for health care practice: A guide to using research evidence.* Philadelphia: W.B. Saunders. 98–124.

Dycoff, D. (2004). Doing it better: Improving practice with a journal club. *Nursing, 34* (7), 29.

Klapper, S. (2001). A tool to educate, critique, and improve practice. *AORN Journal, 74* (5), 712, 714–715.

Pasek, T., & Zack, J. (2004). Cultivating a research milieu: Journal clubs in the pediatric intensive care unit. *Critical Care Nurse, 24* (6), 96–95.

Phillips, R., & Glasziou, P. (2004). What makes evidence-based journal clubs succeed? ACP *Journal Club,* 140, A11–A12. Retrieved January 9, 2006, from *www.acpjc.org/Content/140/3/ issueACPJC-2004-140-3-A11.htm.*

Speers, A.T. (1999). An introduction to nursing research through an OR nursing journal club. *AORN Journal,* 1232, 1235–1236.

Older article, but a classic:

Beck, CT. (1993). Qualitative research: The evaluation of its credibility, fitting-ness, and auditability. *Western Journal of Nursing Research, 15* (2), 263–266.

Older article, but a classic:

Duffy, M.E. (1985). A research appraisal checklist for evaluating nursing research reports. *Nursing & Health Care, 6* (10), 538–547.

Gennaro, S., Hodnett, E., & Kearney, M. (2001). Making evidence-based prac-tice a reality in your institution: Evaluating the evidence and using the evidence to change clinical practice. *The American Journal of Maternal/Child Nursing, 26* (5), 236–45.

Kearney, MH. (2001). Focus on research methods. Levels and applications of qualitative research evidence. Research in Nursing & Health, *24* (2), 145–53.

St. Pierre, J. (2005). Changing nursing practice through a nursing journal club. *MEDSURG Nursing, 14* (6), 390–392.

6

Answering questions with nursing research

Learning objectives

After reading this chapter, the participant should be able to
- identify the role of nursing research in answering questions
- discuss approaches to developing a nursing research project

Overview of research methods

When insufficient quality "evidence" exists to answer a clinical question, nurses might decide to conduct a research study. As nurses become familiar with nursing research studies, they will note that published articles have a logical sequence of events. The research process also includes many of the same elements. Fain (2004) describes a model of the research process that consists of five phases: 1) selecting and defining the problem; 2) selecting a research design; 3) collecting data; 4) analyzing data; and 5) using the findings.

Research methods in nursing cover an entire college course. Many textbooks cover the subject comprehensively (Burns & Grove, 2005; Fain, 2004; Polit & Beck, 2003). Traditionally, nursing research has been categorized as quantitative, qualitative, or some combination of both. Research designs for quantitative research include descriptive, correlational, quasi-experimental, or experimental. The most common research designs for qualitative studies include phenomenology, grounded theory, ethnography, and historical research. Recently, additional types of research, such as outcomes research and intervention research, are being reported more frequently in the nursing literature. Burns and Grove (2005) provide an in-depth resource on these topics.

If you are interested in conducting a research study but do not feel that you have the time, consider teaming up with other nurses and nurse researchers. Collaboration on a research study can be rewarding and is a good way to divide the work (e.g., review of literature, data collection, analyses). Collaboration brings diverse perspectives to the table and results in a better-designed study that produces more reliable and valid results.

Ask a research question

The research question helps determine the methodology that will be used on a given study. Some questions can be answered with quantitative measures such as clinical data. If little is known about a topic or a deep understanding of a phenomenon is desired, then qualitative methods might be more appropriate. Thus, refining the research question is a key step and is not as simple as beginners might imagine. Asking the right question may be difficult, but it is probably one of the most important parts of the research process.

Tips for Success

Want to participate in nursing research, but don't have the time? Team up with other nurses in a collaborative study.

Research questions can come from many places, including personal clinical experience, organizational data, or the professional literature. The question should be important to clinical practice and patient outcomes. It should always be an area of great interest to the researcher so that it is easy to remain committed to and excited about the project during the design, implementation, and analysis phases of the study.

Review pre-existing research

After identifying an area of concern, conduct a thorough review of the literature to determine what research exists related to the question. Many research articles offer suggestions about areas for future research and provide guidance to a researcher in search of a question. In addition, there may be enough evidence available and no need to conduct the study. A review of the literature will also help focus the question.

Consider your specific circumstances

Be sure to consider specific patient populations or experiences as possible focus areas. It is important to ask a question that can be answered by a research project within the constraints of a particular setting and the availability of study subjects.

Nurses, by the nature of their role and close proximity to the patient and patients' families, are in an excellent position to ask questions related to clinical care and patient outcomes. Possible research questions include the following:

- Is there a better way to handle a patient care issue?
- Will the proposed new equipment/technology be more effective?
- Will this new education program for patients increase their satisfaction?

Clinical experiences sometimes lend themselves to further research. For example, when one clinical unit adopted an evidence-based guideline and found that it was not working as expected, the nurses pursued a research project to find out why. When that hospital changed its practice of flushing intermittent peripheral intravenous (IV) catheters from heparin to saline, nurses in the neonatal intensive care unit noticed more problems with occlusion in the very tiny (24-gauge) catheters, which meant that they needed to replace the IV locks more frequently. After reviewing the literature and finding that very few, if any, of the available original research was done with small-bore catheters, they decided to conduct a research study themselves (Mudge, Forcier, & Slattery, 1998).

Another source for inspiration for research questions is from organizational data, such as quality improvement data, or from national data on patient outcomes and patient safety initiatives (discussed in Chapter 8).

The difficulty of designing a research study

Designing a research study that is scientifically rigorous and ethically sound is a complex process well beyond full description in this book. Choosing the correct methodology, selecting valid and reliable instrumentation, establishing proper procedures for data collection, selecting an appropriate sample size, and planning the appropriate statistical analyses require input from an experienced researcher. The research books by Burns and Grove (2005) or Fain (2004) are excellent resources and will help the novice researcher understand the process more thoroughly. They also will provide the tools to help get started.

Develop a research proposal

Once you have formulated your research question, the next step is to develop a proposal. A research proposal is the "roadmap" or "plan" of how you propose to answer your question. It has several components, the format of which may be described or determined by the healthcare organization, a grant-funding agency, or a school program.

The sections of a research proposal consist of the following:

1. Introduction, which includes the problem, its background, and its significance.
2. Review of relevant literature. Identify gaps.
3. Methods and procedures, including
    a. the study design
    b. location of the study
    c. the sample
    d. what will be measured
    e. which instruments will be used
    f. other details of implementing the study
4. Data analysis plan
5. The possible risks and benefits to participants
6. Informed consent procedures, including copies of the informed consent documents
7. Limitations of the proposed study
8. Timeline for the study plan

Introduction and literature review

The researcher must introduce the topic and explain why the problem is significant and worthy of conducting research. Next, he or she must provide a concise, succinct summary of the research and the literature on the topic. These two sections are critical to presenting the research questions, what is known on the topic, and how this research will help build upon or extend current knowledge.

Methodology

Next, the researcher needs to describe fully the methodology of the study. Key components of this section include specifying

- who the subjects/participants will be

- how they will be recruited
- how informed consent will be obtained
- every other step of the research process, including the data-analysis plan

The researcher needs to explain fully how the study will be conducted. The study might include an intervention such as an educational session, completing a survey, or taking physiological measures. The researchers also must describe any benefits or potential risks (physical, psychological, social, legal, or other side effects) to subjects, and how they will be protected. The researcher must describe any potential limitations in the study's design and their effects on research findings. The methodology should include the timeline for implementing the study, should match the study design, and should be explicit about the procedures in the study. This document will become the guidebook for implementing the study, adhering to the protocol, and increasing the reliability of the results.

Words to the wise

When developing the research proposal, note that it is difficult and time-consuming work even for the experienced researcher. For novices learning the research process, it can take even more time. Using a structured format helps any researcher stay organized, so use one that requires both an outline and one that keeps references in an orderly fashion.

Also keep in mind who will be reading the proposal later on. If it is for a school project, tailor the format to criteria set forth by your education program. If it is going to the Institutional Review Board (IRB), use the criteria or guidelines required. If a research proposal is written in response to a request for proposals (RFP), then follow the RFP's directions with exacting detail, making sure the question matches the funding priorities.

Often a proposal contains the same elements as a published research article. The difference between them is that a proposal tells what you plan to do and a published research article describes what was done. A well-written proposal includes enough detail that someone else could follow the procedures exactly.

Have the proposal reviewed

Once a proposal is developed, there are several people and processes involved in a review. All research that involves human subjects, for example, must be approved by an IRB. Some institutions elect to have a peer review process (either through a nursing research council or through a departmental review) in place as a first step, prior to review by the IRB.

Peer review

A peer review of a proposal conducted by either a nursing research committee or some type of departmental review provides the researcher with feedback from a nursing perspective. If a student or a researcher from an outside organization submits a proposal, the researcher will benefit from the knowledge of the organizational culture and systems. The researcher should consider this process a way to enhance any research proposal.

In addition, receiving the input from nurses who have a broad scope of experience and a different perspective on patients and the research process can be very helpful. Any suggestions provided in the peer review will strengthen the proposal before it goes to the Institutional Review Board.

The nursing research council

Nursing research councils (or committees) support nursing research and evidence-based practice efforts of nurses in many clinical settings. Organizational structure, composition, and specific functions vary by organization, but commonly they review the latest research, suggest topics for research projects, provide grant funding if available, and undertake multidisciplinary research projects. Others provide education and consultation to foster evidence-based practice and improve the research knowledge of council members and other staff nurses.

One of a nursing research council's roles is to perform peer review for nursing research study proposals. The council/committee should develop the criteria they will use in their review and provide them to nurse researchers ahead of time. Such criteria should include a brief review of both administrative feasibility and scientific merit (see Figure 6.1: Sample scientific review of research proposals form). The nurse administrator should conduct a more complete review of administrative feasibility on the unit(s) where the study will occur.

Peer review provides the benefit of different perspectives, and in the process of gaining those perspectives, the researcher can strengthen the proposal. This review occurs before submitting the proposal to the IRB of the organization. Some research committees post the nursing research priorities on their Web page to encourage proposals that align with organizational goals.

FIGURE 6.1 **Sample scientific review of research proposals form**

Dartmouth-Hitchcock Medical Center
Lebanon, New Hampshire
Office of Professional Nursing

FORM FOR SCIENTIFIC REVIEW OF RESEARCH PROPOSALS

Project titles: _____
Investigator(s): _____
Affiliation(s): _____
_____

The questions in Part A of this form are to be answered to the best of your knowledge. You do not need to seek out answers that you currently do not possess. This section is only meant to serve as a global feasibility review. A full administrative review will be done by appropriate nursing directors.

A. REVIEW FOR FEASIBILITY

Comments

1. Are the required data and/or subjects available? ( )Yes ( ) No

2. Are the projected dates for data collection reasonable? ( )Yes ( ) No

3. Is the investigator qualified to conduct this study? ( )Yes ( ) No

4. Will the study compromise or interfere with patient care? ( )Yes ( ) No

5. Will the study compromise or interfere with present or
   projected research? ( )Yes ( ) No

6. Is the study consistent with the philosophy, objectives,
   and policies of the Department of Professional Nursing? ( )Yes ( ) No

7. Is the proposed study feasible at DHMC at this time? ( )Yes ( ) No

If there are major obstacles to feasibility, you may stop after completing Part A and return this form to the Nursing Research Coordinator. If there are no obstacles to feasibility, please complete Parts B & C.

B. SCIENTIFIC REVIEW

Comments/Suggested Changes

1. Research problem:
   Is the problem relevant?
   Does the background statement give adequate rationale for study?
   Have appropriate variables been selected?

FIGURE 6.1
Sample scientific review of research proposals form (cont.)

Comments/Suggested Changes

2. Sample:
   Is the method of sample selection appropriate?
   Are the subjects adequate in number and appropriate in type?

3. Procedure:
   Is the research design appropriate to the study?
   Are the procedures to be employed clinically sound?
   Are the tools/measurements appropriate; will they yield the desired data?

4. Risks/Benefits:
   Is the risk-benefit ratio acceptable?
   Are procedures for informed consent adequate?

5. Data analysis:
   Is the data analysis plan adequate for the purpose of this study?

6. Overall evaluation
   (Please rate this proposal on each of the following factors):

	Excellent				Poor
a. importance of the problem addressed	5	4	3	2	1
b. usefulness/applicability of results	5	4	3	2	1
c. overall scientific merit of study	5	4	3	2	1

C. APPROVAL

Please circle one response following each statement:

1. This study has sufficient scientific merit to warrant approval for its conduct within this hospital.

   a. Yes   b. No

2. My level of excitement and support for this project is:

   a. very high
   b. moderately high
   c. neutral
   d. moderately low
   e. very low

Name of reviewer: _____

Date: _____

Send completed review to Nursing Research Coordinator, Office of Professional Nursing.
Source: Dartmouth-Hitchcock Medical Center-Used with permission

Departmental reviews

Organizations that do not have a nursing research committee may undertake a process of peer review within the nursing department. Often the research review is conducted by an ad-hoc group of nurses who are selected for their areas of specialization and experience. They are also qualified to evaluate the scientific merit and administrative feasibility of the study.

Nurses with master's and doctoral education may be best prepared to critique the study proposal for scientific merit and feasibility. For example, a proposal involving breastfeeding in the intensive care nursery might be reviewed by a master's-prepared lactation nurse, the clinical nurse specialist in the intensive care nursery, and a nurse with knowledge or experience in the proposed research methodology.

Institutional Review Board

All research involving human subjects must be reviewed by an IRB, which is a committee whose purpose is to protect the rights of human subjects participating in research studies. The IRB is guided by ethical principles and federal regulations. To learn more about IRBs and federal requirements related to the process, access the following resources:

- Office of Human Research Protection (*www.hhs.gov/ohrp*)
- Office of Human Subject Research (*http://ohsr.od.nih.gov/*)
- Collaborative IRB training initiative *(www.miami.edu/citireg)*

Research proposals are evaluated based on the research complexity, the level of risk for harm, and the vulnerability of the subjects being studied (Lynn & Nelson, 2005). There are three levels of review based on potential risk for harm and complexity: 1) full committee review, 2) expedited review, and 3) exempt from review. The full committee would review studies that have greater risk or whose subjects are considered vulnerable for some reason (e.g., prisoners or pregnant women, when the fetus might be at risk). Studies that are determined to have less than minimal risk (e.g., a study that examined the effect of a group diabetes educational intervention on patients' knowledge level of glucose monitoring techniques) can be reviewed by a sub-group of the committee in an expedited review. Some studies of no risk, of very minimal risk, or in which data are anonymous are determined to be exempt from further review.

The format for submission to the IRB is organization-specific. It should include the complete research proposal, including study design, process for informed consent, risk/benefit assessment, and the selection of subjects. The researcher also should submit any instruments, recruitment materials (posters) and informed consent documents.

Informed consent

The IRB evaluates the informed consent process and related documents closely, and the way in which the information is communicated is as important as the information. For example, certain times would be inappropriate for obtaining informed consent from surgical patients, such as after they have been given pre-operative sedation.

Informed consent is not just a paper that the research subject signs. Rather, it is an ongoing process of communication between the researcher and the subject. Elements of informed consent address the following:

1. Information about the study, including its purpose and what it entails
2. It should be comprehendible (eighth-grade reading level suggested)
3. Potential risk or discomforts
4. Foreseeable benefits
5. Costs to the subject
6. Data confidentiality and how it will be protected
7. That participation is voluntary and that they may choose not to participate or withdraw at any time and without penalty
8. Alternatives to participation

For an example of an informed consent document template, including new additions related to the Health Insurance Portability and Accountability Act of 1996 (HIPAA), see *www.dartmouth. edu/~cphs*.

Collaborating with external researchers

Establishing collaborative relationships with researchers from an outside organization can be mutually beneficial. For example, if you work in a hospital but do not have a nurse researcher to act as a mentor, try collaborating with a nurse researcher from a school of nursing who needs access to a clinical site and who could share his or her research expertise. Some collaborative research takes place with two or more hospitals in which the primary investigator works with the other organization to collect data from a larger patient population than would be available in one organization alone.

For example, if undertaken at one organization, a study that involves a rare event or patient condition would require an unreasonable amount of time to gather a sample that is large enough to be meaningful. Collaborating with researchers from other organizations to conduct a joint project would shorten the time period for subject recruitment and, if well designed, lead to a more valid study.

Involve staff nurses in data collection or data analysis

Involvement in data collection on a study is a helpful way to learn about that part of the research process. For example, in the nursing study of heparin vs. saline mentioned earlier, staff nurses in the neonatal intensive care unit and pediatric unit collected data on a log developed by staff, with the help of a nurse researcher in the institution. One of the staff nurses entered the data into a database and participated in data analyses with the researcher. Involvement in all levels of the project greatly enhanced learning about the research process and enabled the staff group to remain committed for the duration of the study.

If nurses are not ready to conduct research, they can participate in data collection at the point of care. They regularly collect data as part of their practice, but when data are collected as part of a research study, there are additional issues to consider. For example, to ensure the validity of results, data need to be collected and recorded in a consistent and complete way. Variations in instrumentation (e.g., automatic vs. manual blood pressure readings) and technique could skew the results in one direction or another. Therefore, be aware of any research conducted in the practice setting and follow the research protocol.

Routine data collection provides another opportunity for nurses to conduct research in their clinical settings. Many clinically relevant nursing questions can be answered with data contained in the medical record, nurse's flow sheets, and other forms of documentation. Outcomes such as blood pressures, temperatures, and pain medication usage can be obtained when documentation is complete. Teaching nurses about the importance of obtaining and recording data in a reliable and valid manner will help them learn concepts integral to any research project while improving the quality of care.

Dissemination: Publications and presentations

To bridge the research-practice gap, share the results of a completed research project. Start locally with a group of peers by presenting the findings at a staff meeting or at nursing grand rounds. Poster presentations are very effective ways to present the results of the project and may engage others in discussion. Consider presenting the completed research at a national nursing conference. Look for the "Call for Abstracts" in various nursing journals or on the Web page of one of the many specialty organizations.

Once you have organized the results for a poster or presentation, create a manuscript. Decide on the target audience for the article and review some journals appropriate to the topic and audience. The author guidelines for most journals either are found in an issue of the journal or on the journal Web page. References to articles that provide guidance on writing for publication can be found in Burns and Grove (2005).

Creating a research fellowship

To develop the knowledge and skills necessary to conduct clinical research in the acute care setting, nurses need release time away from direct patient care. This requires organizational commitment and may not always be possible in the very busy clinical environment.

Hinds (2000) described the development of a successful nursing research fellowship program in an acute care setting in which a group of 12 staff nurses participated in a 12-month program. The fellowship included one shift per month of protected time with a curriculum that included didactic and skill-building exercises. The faculty consisted of two nurse researchers and many guest lecturers with expertise in research. Fellows were incorporated into protocol-planning sessions and conducted a research study on fatigue in adolescents with cancer. The findings were disseminated through numerous presentations, and short-term organizational outcomes of the program were positive.

Similar to the fellowship described above, Cullen and Titler (2004) described an evidence-based practice staff nurse internship program in acute care. This program was designed to help staff implement and evaluate an evidence-based practice change. Six teams (each composed of a staff nurse, a nurse manager, and an advanced practice nurse) were selected for the 12-month program, which included didactic group discussion and paid clinical release time. The program resulted in positive outcomes for the staff nurses, improved quality of patient care, and six evidence-based practice changes.

Questions that should not be answered by research

Research conducted with the right support can be fun and rewarding. However, it is not always the answer to many of nursing's clinical questions. In fact, some questions should be answered by other methods, including the following:

- Ethical analysis
- Cost-benefit analysis
- Quality improvement
- Program evaluation
- Root cause analysis
- Clinical expertise and scientific principles

Remember that the methods must match the question and the clinical situation (Beyea & Nicoll, 2000). Also, remember that conducting a survey does not equal research (Beyea & Nicoll, 1999). To ensure that your research is valid, work with experts prior to embarking on any project. Ascertain that the methods and processes will help answer the question, and be certain to meet any standards.

Practice exercises

1. Brainstorm with your nursing peers to come up with a list of five clinical issues that would be of interest to you and affect patient care.
2. Identify the resources available in your institution to help you conduct a research study.
3. Read a research study in a nursing journal. Can you identify future topics for research from the article?
4. Examine the methods section in a nursing research article. Can you describe the procedure and instruments the investigator used to collect data?
5. Go to the Web site for the National Institute of Nursing Research (*http://ninr. nih.gov*) Use one of their research priorities to develop a research question for your practice area.

References

Beyea, S. C., & Nicoll, L.H. (1999). A survey does not equal research. *AORN Journal, 69* (1), 263–264.

Beyea, S. C., & Nicoll, L.H. (2000). Decision analysis-putting it all together. *AORN Journal, 71* (3), 678–681.

Burns, N., & Grove, S.K. (2005). *The practice of nursing research: Conduct, critique, and utilization.* (5th ed.) St. Louis: Elsevier Saunders.

Cullen, L., & Titler, M. (2004). Promoting evidence-based practice: An internship for staff nurses. *Worldviews on Evidence-Based Nursing, 1* (4), 215–223.

Fain, J. A. (2004). *Reading, understanding, and applying nursing research.* Philadelphia: F.A. Davis.

Hinds, P., Gattuso, J., & Morrell, A.. (2000). Creating a hospital-based nursing research fellowship program for staff nurses. *Journal of Nursing Administration, 30* (6), 317–24.

Lynn, M. R., & Nelson, D.K. (2005). Common (mis)perceptions about IRB review of human subjects research. *Nursing Science Quarterly, 16* (3), 264–270.

Mudge, B., Forcier, D., & Slattery, M. (1998). Patency of 24-gauge peripheral intermittent infusion devices: A comparison of heparin and saline flush solutions. *Pediatric Nursing, 24* (2), 142–145, 149.

Polit, D. F., & Beck, C.T. (2003). *Nursing research: Principles and methods.* Philadelphia: Lippincott Williams & Wilkins.

Agency for Healthcare Research and Quality. (2005). *Research Priorities for the Agency for Healthcare Research and Quality*. Retrieved January 17, 2006, from http://grants1.nih.gov/grants/guide/notice-files/NOT-HS-06-032.html.

Brink, P. J., & Wood, M. J. (1998). *Advanced design in nursing research*. 2nd ed. London: Sage.

Brink, P. J., & Wood, M. J. (2005). *Basic steps in planning nursing research*. Sudbury, MA: Jones & Bartlett.

Holloway, I., & Wheeler, S. (2002). *Qualitative research in nursing*. Oxford: Blackwell.

Hinshaw, A. S. (2000). Nursing knowledge for the 21st century: Opportunities and challenges. *Journal of Nursing Scholarship, 32* (2): 117–123.

Hinshaw, A. S., Feethan, S. L., & Shaver, J. L. (1999). *Handbook of clinical nursing research*. London: Sage.

Munhall, P. L., & Oiler, C. J. (2001). *Nursing research: A qualitative perspective*. Sudbury, MA: Jones & Bartlett.

Munro, B. H. (2004). *Statistical Methods for Health Care Research*. (5th ed.) Philadelphia: Lippincott Williams & Wilkins.

National Institute of Nursing Research. (2005). Mission Statement. Retrieved on January 17, 2006, from http://ninr.nih.gov.

Waltz, C. F., Strickland, O. L., & Lenz, E. R. (2005). *Measurement in nursing and health research*. New York: Springer.

Nursing excellence and evidence-based practice

Learning objectives

After reading this chapter, the participant should be able to
- describe the relationship of nursing excellence to EBP
- identify approaches to demonstrating the links between EBP, nursing excellence, and the ANCC Magnet Recognition Program® (MRP)

Relationship of nursing excellence to evidence-based practice

Nurses and other clinicians strive to provide the best care possible, and in today's healthcare environment, evidence-based care is an integral component of it. For nurses to achieve excellence, they need resources that support evidence-based care and best practice.

ANCC Magnet Recognition Program®

In the past decade, the Magnet Recognition Program (MRP) has been synonymous with practice environments in which nurses prefer to practice and patients achieve the best outcomes. Much evidence exists that hospitals that attract and retain registered nurses demonstrate key characteristics related to their nurse leader, the professional attributes of staff nurses, and their professional practice environment (Scott, Sochalski, & Aiken, 1999; McClure & Hinshaw, 2002). Additional research supports the benefits of professional practice environments to patients as well as to nursing staff.

Findings also show significant evidence that MRP status hospitals experience decreased mortality rates, lengths of stay, and needle-stick injuries (Aiken, 2002). Other research efforts have reported that higher nurse staffing levels are associated with lower rates of mortality as well as decreased lengths of stay and lower rates of pneumonia, urinary tract infections (Blegen, Goode, & Reed, 1998), and skin breakdown (ANA, 2000). Needleman, Bauerhouse, Mattke, Stewart, and Jalevinsky (2002) reported that higher nurse staffing was associated with decreased rates related to failure to rescue, length of stay, pneumonia, GI bleeding, shock, and cardiac arrest.

If nurse staffing levels serve as the primary characteristic of professional nursing environments, the solution might appear easy. A chief nursing officer could simply hire and try to retain more nurses. There are, however, many other components of a professional practice model. The Magnet Recognition Program identifies and defines the "Forces of Magnetism" as the characteristics displayed by healthcare organizations that develop and maintain a professional practice environment that helps recruit and retain nurses (American Nurses Credentialing Center, 2004). These 14 forces include the following:

- High-quality nursing leadership
- Flat, non-hierarchical organizational structures
- Participative management style
- Personnel policies and programs that support professional nursing practice
- Professional models of care that support nurses' autonomy and accountability
- High-quality patient care
- High levels of nurse participation in quality improvement
- Adequate consultation and human resources
- Nurses practice in an autonomous fashion, consistent with professional practice standards
- The hospital is viewed as a strong, positive, and productive corporate citizen
- Nurses provide teaching in all aspects of their practice
- Nurses are viewed as essential members of the healthcare team
- Positive interdisciplinary relationships exist
- Opportunities and resources exist for professional development across the career trajectory

For a hospital to achieve designation, the environment must support nurses in providing the highest achievable patient outcomes. Thus, a healthcare organization must address all 14 Forces of Magnetism.

ANCC Magnet Recognition Program® and evidence-based healthcare

Evidence-based findings are embedded in each of the Forces. Thus, research guides the Magnet Recognition Program and healthcare organizations in their efforts to provide high-quality care.

To provide excellent care, nurses must have adequate support in their efforts toward continual improvement and their use of research findings. The chief nurse executive must be committed to providing resources that help the nursing leadership team and the staff nurses to implement evidence-based practice. The senior nurse executive also supports efforts to challenge prevailing assumptions and practice standards. Indeed, if you don't create an environment in which the status quo can be questioned, meaningful change based on evidence cannot occur.

Making EBP visible

If a healthcare organization and nursing department values evidence-based practice, they must make those values visible. That is, nurses must see evidence that the organization is committed to using research findings. To do so, organizations must provide the necessary resources, including access to library and electronic resources. Furthmore, an organization must support and create opportunities for nurses to collaborate with a nurse researcher or a nursing faculty member with expertise in nursing research. Additionally, nurses must have time to work on evidence-based projects.

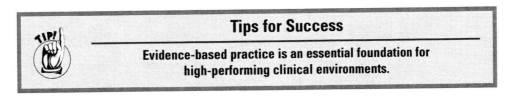

Tips for Success

Evidence-based practice is an essential foundation for
high-performing clinical environments.

Apply EBP to staff satisfaction

Nurse leaders must be willing to use the latest research findings to contribute to management initiatives. They must show a willingness to explore and adopt the best management practices, and the leadership team must strive constantly to improve the practice environment.

For example, an organization's nursing satisfaction surveys might offer evidence that nurses are dissatisfied with rotating shifts. The leadership team can decide to use this evidence in its efforts to improve nurse satisfaction. Changing a staffing and scheduling framework offers its own challenges, but by not addressing this critical issue, a clinical department may suffer from a high turnover rate and may experience lower patient satisfaction scores than other clinical units.

Relying on the premise that "this is the way we have always done it" and ignoring the evidence results in lower performance overall. Addressing the staffing framework up front may save work in the long run related to hiring and orienting new staff members.

Tips for Success

Nurse leaders should use research findings to support management initiatives.

Use evidence to solve everyday problems

The leadership team must be willing and able to pursue evidence-based answers to everyday problems. In the example of rotating shifts, the management team should conduct a literature search and obtain evidence about "best practices" in scheduling nurses. If no specific evidence exists, the management team could collect information from organizations with the lowest turnover rates. The leadership team also could collect specific data from staff nurses about their preferred work hours. This information could be included in an analysis of the unit's daily census, rates of admissions and discharges, or other indicators of department activity.

Sample everyday problem

Many organizations are working to increase their rate of compliance with pneumococcal and flu vaccine administration for patients in hospital and ambulatory settings. These research-based clinical interventions help decrease patient morbidity and mortality. One strategy to increase compliance with them could be to tell the nurses to do a better job of administering these vaccines. Another strategy would be to collect information from the literature and other organizations that have been successful in this initiative. The next step would be to critique the data to find a fit for your specific clinical environment.

From when it begins, the entire initiative must be visible to the front-line caregivers who will administer the vaccines. First, clinicians need to know that giving eligible patients these vaccines is best practice and why. Next, by including staff nurses in the critique of the research and other findings, they are able to contribute to developing a strategy that will result in success. For example, who will remind nurses on inpatient units to administer medications, and how will it be done? Including nurses in the process can ensure that you use effective strategies. Keeping the process visible in this way makes it apparent that nurses are integral to ensuring continuous improvement.

Imagine working in a clinical environment where the nurse leaders simply send a memo that states, "Starting tomorrow, nurses will administer flu vaccine to all eligible patients prior to discharge." It is hard to believe that nurses would comply with this dictate 100% of the time. Nurses might well ask questions:

- Who is going to write the order?
- Why is this the nurses' responsibility?
- How are we going to get this vaccine?
- Isn't this dictate going to delay discharges?
- Can't the vaccination be done at the next office visit?
- How am I going to find time to do this?
- Why are we doing this? Who thought of this idea?

One might wonder whether a professional practice environment exists when decisions are made from the top down, which is not how evidence-based practice occurs. Creating the right environment requires nurses and leaders to use evidence in their efforts to achieve the highest possible outcomes.

The merit of making evidence-based practice visible helps make it a core value within an organization. Evidence-based practice should never be seen as the latest fad or as something that leadership values only for the purpose of seeking designation. If an organization does not fully commit to evidence-based practice, it will not work—not to mention the fact that an organization limits its chances of attaining or maintaining designation.

Tips for Success

EBP should not be adopted as the latest fad. It should
become one of the organization's core values.

ANCC Magnet Recognition Program® and nursing excellence

Many healthcare organizations increase their attention to evidence-based practice when they begin to seek designation. When the chief nurse executive begins the journey, evidence about professional practice environments may guide the journey. Research findings about the best practice environments to recruit and retain nurses while improving patient outcomes may serve as a major objective in the effort.

Chief nurse executives support professional practice environments by integrating evidence into every nursing effort. A nursing organization may have decades of experience with evidence-based practice or may be adopting it as a relatively new strategy. For it to be successful, all clinicians must focus on best practices and ready-to-use evidence. In the pursuit of designation, some nursing organizations believe that having nurses use evidence will be enough to meet or exceed the criteria.

Imagine the following situation, and consider whether it is consistent with the Forces of Magnetism: A team of nurses is concerned about the incidence of bloodstream infections associated with central venous catheters. The concerned nurses work with members of the multidisciplinary team but cannot recruit a physician to participate in the effort. The team members conduct a literature search, critique the research evidence, conduct clinical observations, and develop a new protocol. The group determines that tighter adherence to surgical asepsis during insertion and a different type of site dressing would be instrumental in decreasing bacterial contamination and, thus, infections. These efforts seem consistent with an evidence-based practice model.

When the group attempts to implement the recommended changes, the physicians will not adhere to the recommended practices. Some providers continue to break surgical asepsis during the insertion and apply the dressing they prefer instead of the best dressing based on the evidence. In fact, they tell the nurses, "Evidence-based practice is cookbook medicine. I am the doctor and I know how to do this."

This example seems a little outrageous, but could it, or something similar, happen when nurses recommend change in a particular organization? Many nurses know of instances where it can and does occur. In an organization where professional practice environments are promoted, however, interdisciplinary collaboration is valued and supported alongside evidence-based practice.

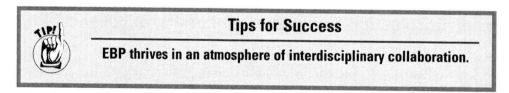

Tips for Success

EBP thrives in an atmosphere of interdisciplinary collaboration.

Support for professional development

When making efforts to promote evidence-based practice and achieve MRP designation, an organization also must address the nursing staff professional development. Limiting professional development to a few continuing education programs on evidence-based practice may not be adequate. An organization also should provide opportunities for nurses to attend conferences or advance their education. Additional resources could include support for nurses to present papers at national or regional meetings.

ANCC Magnet Recognition Program® is more than the 14 Forces of Magnetism—it reflects a synergy of efforts that relate to the Forces and a constant striving toward continual improvement of patient outcomes. To achieve designation and truly make evidence-based practice come alive, demonstrate evidence of synergy between those efforts. Evidence should serve patients, nurses, and the organization in the most effective manner possible.

Providing evidence for designation

When organizations apply for MRP designation, they must provide narratives and sources of evidence related to each of the 14 Forces. An organization must be able to provide evidence of a track record and of ongoing efforts related to each of the Forces. Organizations should consider providing materials about how they use evidence to address each of the 14 Forces. Consider numerous strategies when compiling information about evidence-based efforts.

In an MRP application, an organization must demonstrate its commitment to collect data about key clinical processes and outcomes and to maintain staff satisfaction. An organization must provide adequate resources to support the efforts of clinicians and others in using the data to improve patient care and the work environment. Be cautioned, however, that it cannot just be about nursing data or nursing-sensitive outcomes: It needs to be about the patients who are served within an organization and the entire work force. Providing evidence that an organization has robust systems for collecting, analyzing, and using data is essential to the process.

Secondly, the nursing leadership team must provide supporting evidence that resources exist for research and evidence-based practice. Depending on the size of the facility and number of nurses, the available resources may vary. The culture of a specific organization contributes to determining which resources might be appropriate. For example, an organization may have a nursing librarian off-site, have a consultant librarian available, or have access to electronic resources at the point-of-care. To help in preparing evidence for the application, keep an inventory of your resources so you can describe them adequately in the materials you submit.

Tips for Success

There is no one-size-fits-all method for EBP and MRP designation. Each organization must determine its own best method for integrating EBP.

Documentation of evidence-based practice should be reflected in policies and procedures and meeting minutes. For example, cite in each policy and procedure any research articles that were reviewed and critiqued during their development. Maintain a reference list of articles that have been reviewed for certain quality improvement efforts. Ensure that minutes reflect a discussion of research findings and their thoughtful critique—doing so helps others understand why certain decisions were made and provides another source of evidence.

Remember, however, that there is no "recipe" for evidence-based practice or achieving MRP status. An organization must truly integrate the use of evidence into all of its efforts. Making certain that the strategies fit the culture will help you to succeed.

Document evidence

To help an organization document evidence-based efforts, take advantage of internal publications, whether print or electronic. Featuring stories about evidence-based efforts and nurses' contributions helps inform the public and staff of what you're doing. In this way, patients and families learn about efforts to improve care, and staff members not involved in the projects learn about how evidence can be used. Likewise, nursing newsletters or nursing annual reports can help disseminate information between various clinical units and get additional staff interested in projects.

Presenting papers or posters about evidence-based or research projects at regional or national meetings offers professional development opportunities. Such efforts also help document evidence-based projects. If it would work in your environment, consider featuring various evidence-based projects within the facility. Display posters in public areas, hold a conference and encourage nurses to participate, or highlight these efforts at other meetings.

When organizations embark on evidence-based projects, goals should include possible publication. Do not underestimate the helpfulness of sharing work. Each day on electronic nursing listservs, for example, someone asks how another organization implemented a change or managed certain issues. Therefore, when a group undertakes a systematic process to solve a clinical problem, information about that effort can help guide others. Sharing that work may update others about the latest research findings and provide insight into which strategies were helpful. Furthermore, publications provide documentation that an organization has participated and does participate in evidence-based practice.

Collecting data related to nurse-sensitive quality indicators and benchmarks is another way to document evidence-based projects. A nursing organization may decide to focus evidence-based efforts on improving performance related to these indicators.

Efforts related to various nurse-sensitive outcomes and the use of evidence could be documented in meeting minutes, care protocols, posters, and presentation. For example, a hospital may want to reduce the occurrence of hospital-acquired pressure ulcers. Meeting minutes may include information about how evidence related to prevention was reviewed, critiqued, and integrated into the skin care protocol. That guideline could include references to the latest research findings about treating pressure areas. The team could develop a poster to disseminate information about practice changes for staff nurses throughout the organization. If the team achieves its goal of improving performance, the group could collaborate to develop a manuscript for publication.

Evidence-based practice should be apparent in all aspects of efforts to develop a professional practice environment. If an organization is seeking MRP designation, evidence-based practice should be fully integrated in all initiatives. The written evidence submitted as part of the application should represent those various efforts clearly. Remember, it is just not about nursing—it is about the environment in which nurses practice.

Practice exercises

1. Consider which characteristics of professional nursing practice exist in your clinical settings. Think about each of the Forces of Magnetism. Ask the question, "What gaps exist between what you think is ideal vs. the current status?" Remember that an MRP status hospital does not have to be perfect. Rather, it has to have processes and resources to address concerns and issues.

2. Ask questions and identify opportunities where evidence might address gaps in the professional practice environment. Go to your library resources and see whether you can find some evidence-based strategies that might help close that gap. Learn to ask what evidence exists when practice changes occur.

3. Try to determine which strategies your organization uses to make evidence-based practice visible. Do you know about efforts on other nursing units? If you do not, find out how you would learn more about these and other multidisciplinary efforts.

4. Determine what opportunities exist for nurses in your organization to learn more about evidence-based practice. Also, find out more about opportunities for professional development, such as tuition reimbursement or support for attendance at professional conferences.

5. If your hospital has already received designation, ask to review the most recently submitted supporting evidence. Look for evidence specific to evidence-based practice. Consider how you might become involved in future initiatives.

References

Aiken, L. (2002). Superior outcomes for Magnet hospitals. The evidence base. In M. McClure & A. Hinshaw (Eds.), *Magnet hospital revisited: Attraction and retention of registered nurses* (pp. 61–82). Washington, DC: American Nurses Publishing.

American Nurses Association. (2000). *Nurse staffing and patient outcomes in the inpatient hospital setting.* Washington, DC: American Nurses Association.

American Nurses Credentialing Center. (2004). *The Magnet Recognition Program®.* Silver Spring, MD: American Nurses Credentialing Center.

Blegen, M., Goode, C., & Reed, L. (1998). Nursing staffing and patient outcomes. *Nursing Research, 47* (1), 43–50.

McClure, M. & Hinshaw, A., (Eds.). (2002). *Magnet hospitals revisited: Attraction and retention of professional nurses.* Washington, DC: American Nurses Publishing.

Needleman, J., Bauerhouse, P., Mattke, S., Stewart, M., & Jalevinsky, K. (2002). Nurse staffing levels and the quality of care in hospitals. *The New England Journal of Medicine, 346* (22), 1715-1722.

Scott, J., Sochalski, J., & Aiken, L. (1999). Review of the Magnet hospital research: Findings and implications for professional nursing practice. *Journal of Nursing Administration, 29* (1), 9–19.

Bolton, L. B., & Goodenough, A. (2003). A magnet nursing service approach to nursing's role in quality improvement. *Nursing Administration Quarterly, 27* (4), 344–354.

Havens, D. S. (2001). Comparing Nursing Infrastructure and Outcomes: ANCC Magnet and NonMagnet CNEs Report. *Nursing Economics, 19* (6), 258–266.

Kramer, M., & Schmalenberg, C. E. (2003). Magnet Hospital Staff Nurses Describe Clinical Autonomy. *Nursing Outlook, 51* (1), 13–19.

Laschinger, H. K. S., Almost, J., & Tuer-Hodes, D. (2003). Workplace Empowerment and Magnet Hospital Characteristics. *Journal of Nursing Administration, 33* (7/8), 410–422.

Monarch, K. (2003). Magnet Hospitals Powerful Force for Excellence. *Reflections on Nursing Leadership,* 10–13.

Stewart-Amidei, C. (2003). A Culture of Excellence. *Journal of Neuroscience Nursing, 35* (2), 69.

Examples of evidence-based nursing practice

Learning objectives

After reading this chapter, the participant should be able to
- identify ways to engage nursing staff members in EBP
- describe various examples of EBP projects

Engaging the nursing staff

An organization will integrate evidence-based practice successfully only if it clearly demonstrates the value of using evidence. If changes in practice result in high-quality patient outcomes, being engaged in the process simply becomes the right thing to do.

Engage nursing staff and help them see the benefits of participating by demonstrating how many current practice standards and practices are evidence-based. For example, most nurses learn to perform cardiopulmonary resuscitation (CPR) and provide care during cardiac emergencies using very specific protocols. Nurses may not be aware that recommendations for CPR reflect decades of research to determine the most effective interventions for both airway and cardiac arrests. Adherence to these standards has resulted in the highest achievable outcomes for patients, including survival. These evidence-based recommendations are updated regularly in accordance with the latest research findings—in fact, the American Heart Association updated the CPR guidelines in 2005 (*www. americanheart.org/eccguidelines*). Thus, when individuals are performing CPR, they are providing evidence-based care.

Many other aspects of care are evidence-based as well, but nurses often do not know which interventions are evidence-based and which are opinion-based. Learning to differentiate between the two becomes an important first step. This process can start by encouraging nurses to ask, "What is the evidence for this practice?" Helping nurses see that evidence-based practice serves as the foundation for many aspects of healthcare can help develop champions for the process.

Tips for Success

Garner support by demonstrating how evidence-based practice leads to high-quality patient care.

For example, national recommendations exist from the National Heart, Lung, and Blood Institute for how and when cholesterol and lipid screening should be performed (*www.nhlbi.nih.gov/guidelines/cholesterol/chol_scr.htm*). Any individual undergoing lipid screening would expect to have testing consistent with the latest recommendations. Another example of evidence-based care involves the treatment of acute ischemic stroke (*http://stroke.ahajournals.org/cgi/content/full/36/4/916*). The best-practice recommendations for this condition also can serve as the medical-legal standard, if there is any question about the quality of care. Imagine providing care to a stroke patient without following the guidelines and making every effort to prevent as many adverse outcomes as possible.

Strategies for success

Tips for Success

Successful practice change requires buy-in from all involved.

Clarify the expected positive outcomes

Evidence-based practice can result in more work for nurses and other clinicians, so make sure that everyone understands the positive outcomes associated with practice changes. One such evidence-based change is implementing tight glycemic control protocols including insulin drips and hourly blood glucose testing (Furnary, Zerr, Grunkemeier, & Starr, 1999; Van den Berghe, et al., 2001). To use this important evidence-based protocol successfully, clinicians must understand the positive outcomes associated with it. Presenting research findings about the significant decreases in serious life-threatening infections, shorter hospital stays, and overall morbidity and mortality helps staff members see the value of the changes (Furnary et al., 1999; Van den Berghe et al., 2001). Acknowledging how the workload will change and planning for it effectively will also help. Getting buy-in for evidence-based changes helps promote success and compliance with the practice standards.

Make clinical outcomes visible

Making clinical outcomes visible to clinicians can help improve performance and motivate staff members to engage in evidence-based practice. Many healthcare organizations post graphs and control charts in a conference room on a specific clinical unit. For example, a clinical unit might regularly post a graph with the average blood glucose levels for hospitalized diabetic patients. Doing so allows clinicians to visualize their progress with achieving glycemic control, which helps them strive for success.

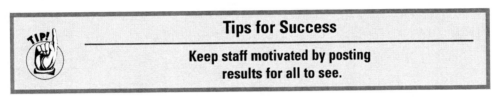

Tips for Success

Keep staff motivated by posting
results for all to see.

Make evidence easy to use

Communicating clearly in written materials will help nurses and others use the information. Therefore, rather than asking nurses to read a complicated new protocol, present the key points initially and then give further details. Focusing on the "need to know" vs. the "nice to know" can help busy clinicians integrate changes in practice.

Re-educate

Present the innovation in a poster or story board format displaying critical information. On a regular basis, reinforce teaching about the changes to remind staff members of facts they may have forgotten. In busy clinical environments where nurses sometimes experience information overload, periodic re-education helps maintain and sustain improvements.

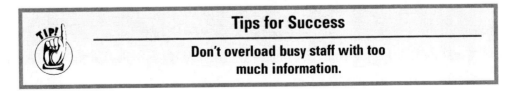

Tips for Success

Don't overload busy staff with too
much information.

Tailor EBP projects to organizational or departmental efforts

In today's healthcare environment, it is essential to create synergies between various efforts. Most acute-care hospitals participate in efforts whose origins rest in evidence-based practice. Nurses, who are active participants in many of these initiatives, are already involved in evidence-based projects.

Three national organizations provide opportunities for nurses to be involved in evidence-based care: the Joint Commission on Accreditation of Healthcare Organizations (JCAHO), the Centers for Medicare & Medicaid Services (CMS), and the Institute for Healthcare Improvement (IHI).

JCAHO-related evidence-based projects

Nurses may work on evidence-based projects related to the JCAHO's National Patient Safety Goals, which creates opportunities for healthcare teams to develop strategies to address these high-priority safety issues, such as

- reducing the risk of patient harm from falls
- reducing the risk of healthcare-associated infections (HAI)

Fall reduction

In 2006, for example, the JCAHO started to require that organizations create fall-reduction programs and evaluate their effectiveness. Most hospitals address this goal in their efforts to maintain JCAHO accreditation and use evidence in the process. Usually, multidisciplinary teams meet to review the evidence and develop a falls prevention and reduction program using the published research, literature, and clinical practice guidelines. Team members critique the published materials and determine the fit to the particular clinical environment. The next steps include disseminating the fall protocol to clinical departments while the multidisciplinary team monitors the overall and department-specific fall rates. Ideally, the group will continue to strive for ongoing improvements in their efforts to reduce and prevent falls using research evidence.

HAI prevention

In terms of preventing healthcare-associated infections, the JCAHO specifically recommends that organizations comply with current Centers for Disease Control and Prevention (CDC) hand-hygiene guidelines. This safety goal offers a perfect opportunity to get involved in evidence-based practice, to collect data, and to improve patient care. In this instance, a multidisciplinary committee could be formed to review the CDC guidelines and to review the organization's current hospital-acquired infection rate. Other activities could include developing a data collection tool and conducting observations of handwashing on various clinical units. The committee could analyze data and plan interventions to increase compliance with the CDC standards. It could design a research project to test which interventions (education, posters, or reminders) are most helpful in increasing compliance. In this way, nurses use evidence-based practice within organizational efforts that are important to high-quality care.

CMS quality initiatives–related EBP projects

Since 2004, CMS has worked with the Hospital Quality Alliance, a national collaboration to encourage hospitals to voluntarily collect and report hospital quality performance information, and to provide a consumer-oriented Web site that reports the data (*www.HospitalCompare.hhs.gov*). This initiative displays data from approximately 4,000 hospitals in the United States. The data compare the quality of care in hospitals based on 20 measures. The current areas of focus include heart attack, heart failure, pneumonia, and the prevention of surgical infections.

For each condition, specific evidence-based outcomes have been identified and defined. For example, in the instance of surgical infection prevention, the following measures have been established:

- Percent of surgery patients who receive preventative antibiotic(s) one hour before incision

- Percent of surgery patients whose preventative antibiotic(s) are stopped within 24 hours after surgery

Each of the measures represents evidence-based best practices for these four conditions. Many healthcare organizations currently focus on improving their performance related to these measures.

This is another opportunity to use evidence to improve practice. Nurses trying to improve performance related to certain measures could conduct a literature and research review. Critiquing the published literature will help nurses understand what interventions might improve performance. This type of public reporting initiative allows nurses to learn how evidence-based practice can contribute to the health of their patients and the success and quality of their organization.

Institute for Healthcare Improvement-related EBP projects

In December 2004, the 100,000 Lives Campaign was launched by the Institute for Healthcare Improvement (IHI). This campaign focuses on six evidence-based healthcare interventions that have been demonstrated to improve patient care and prevent avoidable deaths (*www.ihi.org*). At present, more than 3,000 hospitals have committed to this project. The six key strategies of this effort include

- establishing and deploying rapid response teams
- providing reliable evidence-based care for acute myocardial infarction
- preventing adverse drug events by implementing medication reconciliation
- preventing central-line infections
- preventing surgical-site infections
- preventing ventilator-associated pneumonias

Each of these interventions provides opportunities for nurses and other clinicians to implement evidence-based practice, improve healthcare quality, and save lives. Involving nurses in such efforts gives them a strong understanding of the value of evidence-based practice.

Examples of evidence-based projects

The following contributed narratives provide examples of evidence-based projects. One has been previously published. Both examples demonstrate how staff nurses can improve patient care by implementing evidence-based practice.

Preventing ventilator-associated pneumonia
By Karen Coppin, MSN, RN, CCRN, Southwestern Vermont Medical Center

Ventilator-associated pneumonia (VAP) presents a serious threat and significant complication for patients on ventilator support. It is a leading cause of morbidity and mortality in the intensive care unit (ICU). Occurrences of VAP can increase a patient's length of stay (LOS) by four to nine days and can cost an additional $20,000–$40,000 per episode (American Association of Critical-Care Nurses, 2004).

For staff members at the Southwestern Vermont Medical Center (SVMC) in Bennington, these facts were of grave concern. Despite implementing practice changes in the ICU to reduce VAP, the center's rate of infection was consistently higher than the national benchmark of 5.3 infections per 1,000 ventilator days. **Karen Coppin, MSN, RN, CCRN,** intensive care patient services coordinator, decided to use EBP to address this problem.

Coppin met with members of the Infection Control Department and the respiratory care patient services coordinator to discuss a plan to reduce the VAP rate. The group decided to use the 2003 Centers for Disease Control (CDC) Clinical Practice Guidelines as their guide. (CDC, 2003). To add to the evidence, group members read research articles to help understand the CDC's guidelines.

The group also reviewed SVMC's current practices and compared them to the CDC's guidelines. For example, the guideline recommended that all patients receiving mechanical ventilation should have the head of the bed elevated at a level of 30–45 degrees. Unit-based audits demonstrated that staff members at SVMC were not 100% compliant with this standard of care. To address this gap in practice, a decision was made to provide staff members with a way to measure the bed elevation level accurately in the future.

Coppin also identified an opportunity to educate RNs about the changes in ICU standard of care for ventilated patients during SVMC's annual competency validation day. The planning group set up a station—called Ventilator Management/Reducing Ventilator-Associated Pneumonia—to educate nurses. The goal of the session was to get nurses to demonstrate knowledge of evidence-based strategies for ventilated patients and to describe evidence-based interventions shown to reduce VAP rates. Before visiting the station, nurses read articles and related literature, including a chart displaying SVMC's VAP rates in past quarters compared to the national average. When nurses visited the station, they received education about the rationale for prevention interventions and need for specific changes in the standard of care for ventilator patients.

SVMC's efforts to change the ICU care guidelines led to immediate results. In the first nine months after the implementation, there was not a single VAP incident at the center.

References:

American Association of Critical-Care Nurses. (2004). Practice alert on ventilator associated pneumonia. Retrievd on January 25, 2006, from *www.aacn.org/AACN/practice Alert.nsf/Files/VAPPP/$file/VAP%20Educational%20Programii.ppt.*

CDC Guidelines for Preventing Health-Care Associated Pneumonia. (2003). MMWR Recommendations and Reports. Retrieved on January 25, 2006, *www.cdc.gov/mmwr/ preview/mmwrhtml/rr5303a1.htm.*

Central venous catheters: Preventing air embolism

By Patricia Matula, RN, MSN, Lehigh Valley Hospital, Allentown, PA

One of the most serious complications that can occur in patients with a central venous catheter (CVC) is air embolism. Researchers report that many nurses falsely believe that the incidence of air embolism is extremely rare (Ely et al. 1999; Kim, et al., 1998) but the actual incidence of line-associated air embolism varies from 1 in 3,000 to 1 in 47 in different reports (Orebaugh, 1992).

At Lehigh Valley Hospital in Allentown, PA, patient care specialists began finding case study reports that air embolism was a threat to patients having a CVC removed. These case studies suggested that it was important to focus on using recommended guidelines and paying meticulous attention to detail when discontinuing a CVC. The patient care specialists decided to re-examine existing practice standards and make changes to the existing CVC procedure. The goal of the project was to ensure that clinical practice was consistent with the most current research evidence.

The researchers—**Debra A. Peter, MSN, RN, C,** a patient care specialist; **Carol Saxman, MSN, RN, CCRN,** also a patient care specialist; and **Patricia Matula, RN, MSN,** a nurse specialist—used the Cumulative Index to Nursing and Allied Health Literature (CINAHL) and Medline resources to seek evidence related to

- patient positioning during and after CVC removal
- patient participation during and after CVC removal
- dressing coverage on the exit site

Research findings included recommendations that the patient be placed in a supine position during central line removal, that the patient participate in the removal (e.g., by holding respirations), and that the site be immediately covered following removal to prevent air from entering the vascular system.

Following the in-depth literature review, the researchers collaborated with and obtained materials from advanced practice nurses across the country (Society of Vascular Nursing listserv), physicians, the infection control department staff members, and the online American College of Cardiovascular Nursing "best practice" Web site. The revised proposed procedure was then shared with physicians at Lehigh Valley, who agreed with the changes.

Using the evidence-based information, the researchers revised the procedural steps as indicated. Critical steps were highlighted to heighten awareness to the potential complications of CVC removal. Two additional crucial steps not previously included were added to the revised procedure:

- Having the patient remain in a supine position for 30 minutes following CVC removal
- Maintaining the exit site dressing for 24 hours

The procedure was reviewed and received the required institutional approval by the Lehigh Valley procedure committee. The procedure was then reviewed by the representative nurses, physicians, the safety department, the infection control department, and the risk management department. The reviewed procedure was then presented to and approved by the hospital-wide practice council.

Posters including the revised procedure were distributed to every patient care unit for an RN to review. A case study was incorporated into the content of the poster to engage the staff in the learning process. In addition, the procedural steps specific to CVC removal were incorporated into the RN orientation program, and the competency of CVC removal was added to the RN Orientation Record.

References:

Ely, E., Hite, R., Albert, B., Johnson, M., Bowton, D., & Haponik, E. (1999). Venous air embolism from central venous catheterization: a need for physician awareness. *Critical Care Medicine, 27,* 2113–2117.

Kim, D., Gottesman, M., Forero, A., Han, D., Myers, D., Forlenza, R., et al. (1998). The CVC removal distress syndrome: an unappreciated complication of CVC removal. *The American Surgeon, 64,* 344-347.

Orebaugh, S. (1992). Venous air embolism: clinical and experimental considerations. *Critical Care Medicine, 20,* 1169–1177.

Peter, D. A., & Saxman, C. (2003). Preventing air embolism when removing CVCs: An evidence-based approach to changing practice. *Journal of the Academy of Medical-Surgical Nurses, 12,* (4) 223–228.

Practice exercises

1. Find out about the evidence-based projects at your healthcare organization and how nurses may be participating. Talk to nurses who are involved and learn more about their efforts. Try to determine whether the latest policy update in your clinical department includes references to research articles or evidence-based articles or guidelines.

2. Visit *www.jcaho.org* and learn more about the National Patient Safety Goals and the Sentinel Event Program. If your organization has JCAHO accreditation, go to *www.jcaho.org/quality+check/index.htm* and learn more about what information is available to the public. Learn more about your organization's activities to address the patient safety goals.

3. Visit *www.HospitalCompare.hhs.gov* and compare the performance of hospitals in your area. Consider how performance varies across settings, and ponder whether the reports you are viewing would contribute to a decision about where an individual might seek healthcare. Find out what your organization is doing to improve performance related to these outcomes.

4. Visit *www.ihi.org* and learn more about the 100,000 Lives Campaign. Read more about one of the initiatives, and consider any gaps between what you learned in school and the current recommendations for practice.

5. Learn about the priorities of your organization and department. Determine which ones are evidence-based, and consider how care can be improved by using the latest research findings.

References

Furnary, A. P., Zerr, K. J., Grunkemeier, G. L., & Starr, A. (1999). Continuous intravenous insulin infusion reduces the incidence of deep sternal wound infection in diabetic patients after cardiac surgical procedures. *Annals of Thoracic Surgery, 67,* 352–362.

Van den Berghe, G., Wouters, P., Weekers, F., Verwaest, C., Bruyninckx, F., Schetz, M., et al. (2001). Intensive insulin therapy in critically ill patients. *New England Journal of Medicine, 345,* 1359–1367.

Further reading

Gagan, M., & Hewitt-Taylor, J. (2004). Professional issues. The issues for nurses involved in implementing evidence in practice. *British Journal of Nursing, 13* (20), 1216–1220.

Gerrish, K., & Clayton, J. (2004). Promoting evidence-based practice: An organizational approach. *Journal of Nursing Management, 12* (2), 114–23.

Krugman, M. (2003). Evidence-based practice: The role of staff development. *Journal for Nurses in Staff Development, 19* (6), 279–287.

Newhouse, R., Dearholt, S., Poe, S., Pugh, LC., & White, KM. (2005). Evidence-based practice: A practical approach to implementation. *Journal of Nursing Administration, 35* (1), 35–40.

Sanares, D., & Heliker, D. (2002). Implementation of an evidence-based nursing practice model: disciplined clinical inquiry. *Journal for Nurses in Staff Development, 18* (5), 233–240

Udod, SA., & Care, WD. (2004). Innovation in leadership. Setting the climate for evidence-based nursing practice: What is the leader's role? *Canadian Journal of Nursing Leadership, 17* (4), 64–75.

Target audience

Chief Nursing Officers

Directors of Nursing

Nurse Managers

HR Professionals

CFO/CEO

Statement of need

Evidence-based practice in nursing has grown out of evidence-based medicine. More organizations are adopting EBP within their nursing departments, but nurses need to know where to go to get the start-up information. This book provides nurses who are new to EBP with information to begin implementing EBP in nursing practice. It explains EBP, identifies internal and external resources, and discusses how to get started. After reading this book, the reader will be able to develop and implement evidence-based nursing practice at his or her facility, which will in turn improve outcomes, patient care, and satisfaction.

Educational objectives

Upon completion of this activity, participants should be able to do the following:

- Define evidence-based practice (EBP)

- Differentiate between evidence-based practice, research, research utilization, and quality improvement

- Describe the importance of EBP to nursing practice and high-quality patient care

- Identify strategies to establish a culture for inquiry and EBP

- Discuss approaches for nurses to participate in EBP and research

- Describe approaches to finding pertinent and reliable literature and research

- Discuss approaches to appraising the strength of the evidence

- Identify a model of EBP

- Discuss approaches to integrate evidence into nursing practice

- Identify why journal clubs are an effective way to start EBP

- Establish guidelines for successful journal clubs

- Identify the role of nursing research in answering questions

- Discuss approaches to developing a nursing research project

- Describe the relationship of nursing excellence to EBP

- Identify approaches to demonstrating the links between EBP and nursing excellence and the ANCC Magnet Recognition Program® (MRP)

- Identify ways to engage nursing staff members in EBP

- Describe various examples of EBP projects

Authors

Suzanne C. Beyea, RN, PhD, FAAN, and Mary Jo Slattery, RN, MS

Accreditation/designation statement

This educational activity for three contact hours is provided by HCPro, Inc. HCPro is accredited as a provider of continuing nursing education by the American Nurses Credentialing Center's Commission on Accreditation.

Disclosure statements

Suzanne C. Beyea and Mary Jo Slattery have declared that they have no commercial/financial vested interest in this activity.

Instructions

In order to be eligible to receive your nursing contact hour(s) for this activity, you are required to do the following:

1. Read the book
2. Complete the exam
3. Complete the evaluation
4. Provide your contact information in the space provided on the exam and evaluation
5. Submit the exam and evaluation to HCPro, Inc.

Please provide all of the information requested above and mail or fax your completed exam, program evaluation, and contact information to

HCPro, Inc.
Attention: Continuing Education Department
200 Hoods Lane
P.O. Box 1168
Marblehead, MA 01945
Fax: 781/639-0179

If you have any questions, please contact our customer service department at 877/727-1728.

Nursing education exam

Name: _____

Title: _____

Facility name: _____

Address: _____

Address: _____

City: _____ State: _____ ZIP: _____

Phone number: _____ Fax number: _____

E-mail: _____

Nursing license number: _____

(ANCC requires a unique identifier for each learner)

1. A definition of evidence-based practice is

    a. providing all patients with the same type of research-based care.

    b. the judicious use of research in the context of the clinician's expertise and patient's desires.

    c. using an evidence-based protocol for a population of patients regardless of their situation.

    d. researching every patient and collecting data to determine what is best for their situation.

2. Which of the following is a characteristic of evidence-based practice?

    a. It is research utilization with a new label.

    b. It is a combination of quality improvement and research.

    c. It involves conducting clinically useful research.

    d. It is the use of research findings to determine best practices.

3. Evidence-based practice is important because

    a. it is a JCAHO requirement for accreditation for our next review.

    b. a hospital needs to do it if it wants to receive ANCC Magnet Recognition®.

    c. it provides a framework to integrate research findings and to provide best practice.

    d. it is the only way to make sure that patients receive the best care.

4. Which of the following statements best represents the relationship between evidence-based practice and other organizational initiatives?

   a. They are parallel processes that rarely intersect and connect.

   b. Evidence and data should guide key initiatives and efforts.

   c. Occasional connections occur in which evidence might help guide efforts.

   d. Organizational initiatives are about leadership, and evidence-based practice is about clinical issues.

5. One way to create a culture for evidence-based practice is by

   a. requiring nurses to participate in journal clubs.

   b. making research classes mandatory.

   c. insisting that nurses read research journals.

   d. assessing the readiness of the organization.

6. One way for nurses to participate in evidence-based practice is through

   a. joining nursing research councils.

   b. returning to school for further education.

   c. hearing about the chief nursing officer's area of clinical expertise.

   d. wearing a button on EBP day.

7. A helpful, fast, and free way to conduct a search of the literature and research is to

   a. visit the library and use the print indexes to identify articles.

   b. search resources on the National Library of Medicine Web site.

   c. ask other nurses for help.

   d. visit the library and search copies of the print journals.

8. The term "strength of the evidence" refers to

   a. how many articles one finds on the topic.

   b. the research methods used in the studies.

   c. whether you believe the research findings.

   d. whether the research fits to clinical practice.

9. Which of the following is NOT a characteristic of the Iowa Model of Evidence-Based Practice?

   a. Knowledge- and problem-focused triggers.

   b. Key decision points.

   c. Sequential, directional processes.

   d. A framework for rating the strength of the research.

10. Which of the following is NOT a strategy to successfully promote integration of evidence into nursing practice?

   a. Including research findings in policies and procedures.

   b. Providing education to nursing staff members.

   c. Requiring all nurses to participate in some type of research activity.

   d. Identifying research champions for each clinical department.

11. Journal clubs are an effective way to begin implementing EBP in an organization because

   a. they provide staff nurses with exposure to research and a chance to discuss it.

   b. management requires staff to participate in journal clubs.

   c. they teach staff nurses clinical skills.

   d. they develop policy and procedures.

12. A successful journal club for nurses depends on the

   a. availability of a nurse researcher to lead the discussion.

   b. availability of the chief nurse executive to lecture the group.

   c. willingness of the group to learn and the availability of a facilitator.

   d. detailed research evaluation form designed for each article.

13. Which of the following statements best describes the nursing research process?

   a. It is only important at hospitals seeking MRP designation.

   b. Properly conducted, it can provide helpful answers.

   c. It should be conducted prior to performing a literature search.

   d. Most nursing research does not require an IRB review.

14. Nursing research should focus on

    a. questions that medical research can't answer.

    b. clinically pertinent questions of concern to nurses.

    c. questions about the education of nurses.

    d. problems focused on developing nursing theories.

15. Which of the following is not a designation for a research protocol by an Institutional Review Board (IRB)?

    a. Exempt

    b. Expedited

    c. Effective

    d. Full committee review

16. The primary purpose of an IRB is to ensure that

    a. researchers follow their guidelines.

    b. scientific methods are reliable and valid.

    c. the rights of human subjects are protected.

    d. funding is not lost through violation of federal guidelines.

17. Nursing excellence and evidence-based practice are

    a. two different concepts and processes.

    b. two interrelated processes, each dependent on the other.

    c. not important to achieving ANCC Magnet Recognition.

    d. JCAHO standards and thus practice requirements.

18. A strategy to help an organization striving to achieve designation and implement evidence-based practice is to

    a. replicate the exact efforts of another organization.

    b. start by adding research references and evidence to policies.

    c. develop strategies that fit the culture of the organization.

    d. expect all staff nurses to undertake EBP projects.

19. A strategy that can help engage staff in evidence-based practice is

    a. sharing information about outcomes and performance indicators.

    b. issuing a memo dictating new practices without including reasons why the old method is being changed.

    c. requiring that each nurse regularly read an academic journal on best practices.

    d. providing detailed and complete protocols to increase understanding.

20. A suitable topic amenable to evidence-based practice is

    a. development of no-lift beds.

    b. investigating environmental factors related to incidence of childhood cancers.

    c. determining nurses' preferred footwear.

    d. prevention of bloodstream infections.

Nursing education evaluation

Name: _____

Title: _____

Facility name: _____

Address: _____

Address: _____

City: _____ State: _____ ZIP: _____

Phone number: _____ Fax number: _____

E-mail: _____

Nursing license number: _____

(ANCC requires a unique identifier for each learner)

1. This activity met the following learning objectives:

Defined evidence-based practice (EBP)

Strongly disagree   1   2   3   4   5   Strongly agree

Differentiated between evidence-based practice, research, research utilization, and quality improvement

Strongly disagree   1   2   3   4   5   Strongly agree

Described the importance of EBP to nursing practice and high-quality patient care

Strongly disagree   1   2   3   4   5   Strongly agree

Identified strategies to establish a culture for inquiry and EBP

Strongly disagree   1   2   3   4   5   Strongly agree

Discussed approaches for nurses to participate in EBP and research

Strongly disagree   1   2   3   4   5   Strongly agree

Described approaches to finding pertinent and reliable literature and research

Strongly disagree   1   2   3   4   5   Strongly agree

Discussed approaches to appraising the strength of the evidence

Strongly disagree   1   2   3   4   5   Strongly agree

Identified a model of EBP

Strongly disagree   1   2   3   4   5   Strongly agree

Discussed approaches to integrate evidence into nursing practice

Strongly disagree   1   2   3   4   5   Strongly agree

Identified why journal clubs are an effective way to start EBP

Strongly disagree   1   2   3   4   5   Strongly agree

Established guidelines for successful journal clubs

Strongly disagree   1   2   3   4   5   Strongly agree

Identified the role of nursing research in answering questions

Strongly disagree   1   2   3   4   5   Strongly agree

Discussed approaches to developing a nursing research project

Strongly disagree   1   2   3   4   5   Strongly agree

Described the relationship of nursing excellence to EBP

Strongly disagree   1   2   3   4   5   Strongly agree

Identified approaches to demonstrating the links between
EBP and nursing excellence and the ANCC Magnet Recognition Program®

Strongly disagree   1   2   3   4   5   Strongly agree

Identified ways to engage nursing staff members in EBP

Strongly disagree   1   2   3   4   5   Strongly agree

Described various examples of EBP projects

Strongly disagree   1   2   3   4   5   Strongly agree

2. Objectives were related to the overall purpose/goal of the activity

Strongly disagree 1   2   3   4   5   Strongly agree

3. This activity was related to my nursing activity needs

Strongly disagree 1   2   3   4   5   Strongly agree

4. The exam for the activity was an accurate test of the knowledge gained

Strongly disagree 1   2   3   4   5   Strongly agree

5. The activity avoided commercial bias or influence

Strongly disagree 1   2   3   4   5   Strongly agree

6. This activity met my expectations

Strongly disagree 1   2   3   4   5   Strongly agree

7. Will this learning activity enhance your professional nursing practice?

   Yes

   No

8. This educational method was an appropriate delivery tool for the nursing/clinical audience

Strongly disagree 1   2   3   4   5   Strongly agree

9. How committed are you to making the behavioral changes suggested in this activity?

   a) Very committed

   b) Somewhat committed

   c) Not committed

10. Please provide us with your degree

   a) ADN

   b) BSN

   c) MSN

   d) Other, please state

11. Please provide us with your credentials
    a) LVN
    b) LPN
    c) RN
    d) NP
    e) Other, please state

12. The fact that this product provides nursing contact hours influenced my decision to buy it
Strongly disagree   1   2   3   4   5   Strongly agree

13. I found the process of obtaining my continuing education credits for this activity easy to complete
Strongly disagree   1   2   3   4   5   Strongly agree

14. If you did not find the process easy to complete, which of the following areas did you find the most difficult?
    a) Understanding the content of the activity
    b) Understanding the instructions
    c) Completing the exam
    d) Completing the evaluation
    e) Other, please state:

15. How much time did it take for you to complete this activity (including reading the book and completing the exam and the evaluation)? _____

16. If you have any comments on this activity, process, or selection of topics for nursing CE, please note them below.

17. Would you be interested in participating as a pilot tester for the development of future HCPro nursing education activities?
Yes
No

Thank you for completing this evaluation of our nursing CE activity.